Everything You Need to Know

About Cancer*

Matthew D. Galsky, MD
Director, Phase I Clinical Trials Program
Comprehensive Cancer Centers of Nevada
Las Vegas, Nevada

*IN LANGUAGE YOU CAN ACTUALLY UNDERSTAND

JONES AND BARTLETT PUBLISHERS
Sudbury, Massachusetts
BOSTON   TORONTO   LONDON   SINGAPORE

World Headquarters
Jones and Bartlett Publishers
40 Tall Pine Drive
Sudbury, MA 01776
978-443-5000
info@jbpub.com
www.jbpub.com

Jones and Bartlett Publishers
Canada
6339 Ormindale Way
Mississauga, Ontario L5V 1J2
Canada

Jones and Bartlett Publishers
International
Barb House, Barb Mews
London W6 7PA
United Kingdom

Jones and Bartlett's books and products are available through most bookstores and online booksellers. To contact Jones and Bartlett Publishers directly, call 800-832-0034, fax 978-443-8000, or visit our website, www.jbpub.com.

Substantial discounts on bulk quantities of Jones and Bartlett's publications are available to corporations, professional associations, and other qualified organizations. For details and specific discount information, contact the special sales department at Jones and Bartlett via the above contact information or send an email to specialsales@jbpub.com.

The authors, editor, and publisher have made every effort to provide accurate information. However, they are not responsible for errors, omissions, or for any outcomes related to the use of the contents of this book and take no responsibility for the use of the products and procedures described. Treatments and side effects described in this book may not be applicable to all people; likewise, some people may require a dose or experience a side effect that is not described herein. Drugs and medical devices are discussed that may have limited availability controlled by the Food and Drug Administration (FDA) for use only in a research study or clinical trial. Research, clinical practice, and government regulations often change the accepted standard in this field. When consideration is being given to use of any drug in the clinical setting, the healthcare provider or reader is responsible for determining FDA status of the drug, reading the package insert, and reviewing prescribing information for the most up-to-date recommendations on dose, precautions, and contraindications, and determining the appropriate usage for the product. This is especially important in the case of drugs that are new or seldom used.

Production Credits

Executive Publisher: Christopher Davis
Senior Editorial Assistant: Jessica Acox
Production Director: Amy Rose
Associate Production Editor: Melissa Elmore
Senior Marketing Manager: Barb Bartoszek
Manufacturing and Inventory Control Supervisor: Amy Bacus
Composition: Northeast Compositors, Inc.
Interior Images: Jay Howell
Printing and Binding: Malloy, Inc.
Cover Printing: Malloy, Inc.

Library of Congress Cataloging-in-Publication Data

Galsky, Matthew D.
Everything you need to know about cancer in language you can actually understand / Matthew D. Galsky.
   p. cm.
Includes index.
ISBN-13: 978-0-7637-6454-8
ISBN-10: 0-7637-6454-X
1. Cancer--Popular works. I. Title.
RC263.G35 2010
616.99'4--dc22

                            2009012328

6048
Printed in the United States of America
13 12 11 10 09   10 9 8 7 6 5 4 3 2 1

This book is for Alan and Eunice Galsky.

CONTENTS

Whenever I see a patient newly diagnosed with cancer for an initial consultation, prior to discussing prognosis or the risks and benefits of treatment, I like to start by explaining what cancer is. Each time I have this conversation, the responses are similar: "I had no idea," or "No one ever explained it to me like that before." In this era of 15-minute doctor visits caused by physician time pressure, the basics of cancer are often ignored in favor of saving time for complex treatment discussions. However, I can't imagine expecting patients (and their families) to sort through their treatment options without understanding the basics.

Fighting cancer is a true battle. To engage successfully in any battle, a plan of attack is needed. This plan of attack is based on gathering intelligence, comparing different strategies, and selecting a strategy that is thought to be most effective while doing the least collateral damage. Like Sun Tzu wrote in *The Art of War*, "Know your enemy."

This book is not a 500-page encyclopedic guide to the diagnosis and management of every form of cancer; nor is it a book of secrets about how to beat cancer with diet or supplements. There are plenty of those books on the shelves. This is a simple, concise manual that explains the very basics of cancer and cancer treatment in language you can understand. This is a book for patients who are newly diagnosed (and their friends and families) and for patients who have been battling cancer who may want a better understanding of their "enemy." My hope is that this will be an easy cover-to-cover read and will provide patients, friends, family, and anyone interested in current health issues with the foundation to understand cancer and cancer treatment. This book is for you.

—Matthew D. Galsky, MD

ACKNOWLEDGMENTS

I would like to thank my wife and my sons for their support and for allowing me the time to complete this book.

CHAPTER 1

So, what is cancer, anyway?

Cancer is a terrifying word—it shakes most of us to our very core. Our parents and grandparents couldn't even say the word; instead, it was the "big C" or not mentioned at all. Despite all of the advances in the diagnosis and treatment of cancer over the past several decades, there is still a lack of general understanding about cancer. Sure, the evening news might report on the latest cancer drug to be approved by the Food and Drug Administration (FDA) or the benefits of eating the berry *du jour* in decreasing cancer risk, but little time is spent explaining what cancer *is*. This book will take you on a journey . . . a journey to demystify cancer. By truly understanding what cancer is, how it develops, and how it is diagnosed and managed, you will be in a much better position to understand the rationale for current cancer treatments and to weigh these treatment options for your family, your friends, or yourself.

It all starts with a single cell. Cells are the building blocks of your organs. Every organ in your body—your heart, lung, brain, bones, intestines, you name it—is made up of hundreds of thousands of tiny cells. These cells are so tiny, in fact, that more than 70,000 could fit on the head of a pin. Even your blood, which is part liquid, is also composed of a host of different cells (more on that later).

Unlike other building blocks in your life, such as the bricks or lumber that make up your house, the job of a cell is much more complex than just providing scaffolding or support. Cells are complex little machines. Each cell has the ability to react to its environment, to communicate with other cells in the same organ, and to communicate with cells in other organs. Cells even

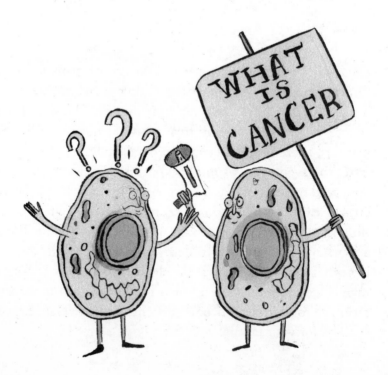

have the ability to repair themselves if they are damaged. Imagine if the bricks in your house could do that—you would save a bundle on homeowner's insurance!

One of the most amazing things about your cells is that although they make up organs that look very different from each other, feel different, and perform vastly different functions, all of the one trillion cells in your body are derived from a single cell called the *fertilized zygote*, the cell formed at the time of your conception. Although scientists don't fully understand how a cell decides to become a heart cell, or a bone cell, or a brain cell, it is known that each cell, regardless of where it ends up, contains the same set of genetic material called deoxyribonucleic acid (DNA). You can think of DNA as the cell's instruction manual. This instruction manual tells a cell where it should go and what kind of cell it should be and even how to perform all of its required functions. A heart cell has the same instruction manual as a bone cell; however, each uses only the specific sections in the manual necessary to perform the job of the organ in which it resides.

If DNA is your cells' instruction manual, then genes are the individual chapters. A *gene* is a small piece of DNA that instructs a cell to make a protein that performs a particular task. Proteins perform all kinds of important jobs in your cells: there are proteins involved in sending signals to other cells and proteins involved in receiving those signals, proteins involved in responding to changes in a cell's environment, proteins involved in cleaning up the "trash" inside of a cell, and on and on. It is easy to imagine how damage to DNA might interfere with production of a particular protein and cause things to go haywire. Think about trying to put together a do-it-yourself bookshelf when one of the chapters in the instruction manual is missing or the pages are stuck together—your bookshelf might come out looking more like a dining room table!

Most of the cells in your body duplicate themselves continuously in a process called *mitosis*. This process is necessary because the cells in your body have a fixed life span, and after doing their job they self-destruct. Your cells also self-destruct if they have been irreversibly damaged. This process of self-destruction is known as *apoptosis*. By cells replicating, your body ensures that you have a sufficient number of cells so that when some self-destruct, there are others to take their place. Your body does this automatically, and constantly, so that you can go about your life, working, eating, sleeping, and not having to worry about whether your liver or your intestines have enough cells to function properly.

Each time a cell duplicates itself, it copies its entire DNA (instruction manual) so that each new cell also has a copy. Surprisingly, this is a highly efficient process, better than, for example, the newest high-tech photocopier with all the bells and whistles. It is estimated that for some types of cells, this process occurs more than 100 billion times a day! Like any process that involves duplication (think of the game telephone you played as a child, where one child whispered a message to the next in succession, and by the end, the message was entirely garbled), with an increased number of copies comes an increased risk that errors will be made. Even the fancy photocopier with all the bells and whistles gets jammed sometimes, or the ink smudges, and not all of the copies turn out perfect. Well, your cells occasionally make errors, too, when copying DNA. These errors are commonly called *mutations*. Fortunately, each cell has an intricate system to repair these errors so that the copies are corrected before they are passed on to the new cells. If the error can't be corrected, then the cell self-destructs. How's that for a complex little machine!

Sometimes the DNA in a cell acquires an error (mutation) that hasn't been repaired and that slips past the self-destruction process. These errors typically have to do with genes (chapters in the instruction manual) that contain information about the duplication or self-destruction process itself. For instance, if an error occurs in the gene that tells the cell when it should self-destruct, then the cell could keep growing and dividing indefinitely without destroying itself because it does not have the proper instructions on the self-destruction process. The abnormal gene is passed on to all of the daughter cells, which continue to grow and divide and pass on the abnormal gene. (Daughter cells are the cells formed by replication of an original cell.) You could imagine if all of these cells were growing and dividing and not dying; they would accumulate and cause a collection of abnormal cells. This collection of abnormal cells is commonly referred to as a *tumor*. Aha! This is the first hallmark of cancer: cells that have gained the ability to duplicate uncontrollably, without self-destructing, and as a result accumulate to form masses or tumors.

Think about the high-tech photocopier. An error in the circuitry could result in copies being made uncontrollably and could prevent the machine from shutting off. Soon, the small office where the copier is located would be overtaken by hundreds and hundreds of copies of the original item. Sounds like an episode of *I Love Lucy*. Similarly, tumor cells growing uncontrollably can start to take over the limited space in the organ in which they reside, and they can start to interfere with the normal function of that organ.

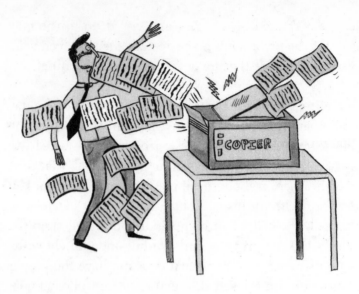

In most cases, scientists don't understand how or why these errors occur in a cell's DNA. Some exposures in the environment might likely predispose cells to acquiring these errors. These exposures include radiation, cigarettes, and certain chemicals, among other things. Infections with certain viruses or bacteria have been linked to the development of specific cancers. (For example, human papillomavirus infection is associated with cervical cancer.) Some families even pass on an error in a specific gene from generation to generation. Remember, all of your cells are descendents of the fertilized zygote, the cell formed at the time of your conception. That means that half of the DNA in your cells originally came from your mother and half from your father—if there was an error in your mother's or father's DNA, there is a chance that it could end up in your DNA as well.

More than one error in the instruction manual is generally required to cause cancer. However, as people age, the chance of acquiring additional errors increases. So, if someone is born with one error already present, then it is that much more likely that a second or third cancer-causing mutation will occur during that person's lifetime. You might have heard of the families that pass on the *BRCA* gene mutation. This is an abnormal gene that is passed on from generation to generation and that carries a significantly increased risk of developing breast cancer and ovarian cancer.

Although a number of hereditary cancer syndromes exist, most cancers are not hereditary. The errors that occur in the DNA that cause most cancers are not *germ line mutations*—that is, the mutations occur in a cell in the organ where the cancer arises, not in the DNA of the cells that form the fertilized zygote. Therefore, these mutations are not passed on to future generations.

The second hallmark of cancer has to do with cells respecting their boundaries. With the exception of the blood cells, discussed in Chapter 2, most normal cells don't leave their organ of origin—this would be like one of the bricks in your house leaving the front porch, traveling down the street, and becoming part of your neighbor's front porch. Similarly, a normal cell in your colon would never leave your colon, and a normal cell in your kidney would never leave your kidney. However, as cancer cells divide and grow, they can gain access to the lymphatic system (sort of like the body's sewer system) or the bloodstream and spread to other parts of the body. When cancer cells spread from their original organ to other parts of the body, they are called *metastases*, or metastatic cancer. The cancer cells can then "set up shop" in these other organs and start duplicating and accumulating, forming masses or tumors at each of these new sites as well.

Think again of the high-tech photocopier, which, of course, has a built-in fax machine. This time, the circuitry malfunction not only leads to hundreds and hundreds of copies being made, cluttering the entire office, but now these copies are also faxed to every other office in the building. You can see how cancer starts as a local problem but often becomes a systemic problem.

Let us review what you have learned so far. (See **Table 1-1** for a list of terms related to cancer and their definitions.) Your organs (and blood) are made up of cells. These cells are in a constant state of duplication and self-destruction to maintain an equilibrium of healthy cells to populate your organs. Each cell has an intricate instruction manual known as DNA, which is copied each time your cells duplicate themselves. The chapters in the instruction manual, the genes, tell your cells which proteins to make to perform various functions. Errors (mutations) can occur in your genes when your DNA is being duplicated. Most of these mutations are repaired; otherwise, the cell self-destructs. Sometimes mutations slip past the repair or duplication process and this allows the affected cell to duplicate uncontrollably. These mutations are passed on to all of the daughter cells, which also duplicate uncontrollably. Soon, there is a collection of abnormal cells that are growing and dividing, and these cells accumulate to form a mass, or tumor. As these cells grow, some can gain access to the bloodstream or the lymphatic system, metastasize (spread) to other organs in the body, and continue this process in a whole new location. This is cancer.

Table 1-1 Some (Often Confusing) Cancer Definitions

Benign tumor   Collection of cells growing abnormally, locally, without the ability to spread to other areas of the body.
Cancer   Malignant tumor.
Carcinoma   Cancers arising from the cells that line the cavities and surfaces of structures throughout the body. Different subtypes of carcinoma depend on the specific cell type involved in a particular location of the body. Adenocarcinomas are cancers originating from glandular tissue. Adenocarcinomas are the most common subtype of cancers arising from organs such as the prostate or colon. Squamous cell carcinomas are the most common subtype of cancers arising from the cervix or the throat.
Leukemia   Cancers arising from blood cells produced by the bone marrow.
Lymphoma   Cancers arising from a subtype of white blood cells, called lymphocytes, that make up the lymph nodes.
Malignant tumor   Collection of cells growing abnormally with the ability to spread to others areas of the body.
Mass   A descriptive term for a "lump" of abnormal tissue detectable on examination of a patient or on an imaging test (for example, a CT scan). A mass may or may not be related to cancer.
Metastasize   Spread of cancer cells to other areas of the body.
Sarcoma   Cancers arising from the cells that make up the supportive structures in the body such as the bone, cartilage, and muscle.
Tumor   An accumulation of cells growing abnormally.

CHAPTER 2

What is the bone marrow, and why is it important in cancer?

As mentioned in the Chapter 1, even your blood is made up of cells. You are probably thinking, how do the cells get into the blood and what is their purpose? Inside every bone in your body is an incredible organ called the bone marrow. The bone marrow is a blood-cell-producing factory. It is constantly churning out new blood cells and releasing them into the bloodstream. The bone marrow makes three major types of cells:

White blood cells: White blood cells are commonly referred to as infection-fighting cells. When these cells are decreased in number in the blood, or when they are not functioning normally, you are at increased risk of developing infections.

Red blood cells: Red blood cells are the cells that carry oxygen from your lungs to all of the other parts of your body. When these cells are decreased in number in your blood, the condition is referred to as *anemia*. Anemia manifests as fatigue, shortness of breath, lightheadedness—all the symptoms you might expect if your body is not getting enough oxygen. Think of anemia as a car running on near empty.

Platelets: Platelets are the cells that keep you from bleeding excessively if you injure yourself. When you form a scab after you get cut, that is your platelets in action. When your platelets are decreased, you are more susceptible to bleeding.

Why would your white blood cells, red blood cells, or platelets ever be decreased in your bloodstream if the factory, the bone marrow, is constantly making new cells? There are several possible reasons why, but for the purposes of this discussion, let's focus on two major (but very different) reasons why the factory might shut down: (1) cancers that originate in the bone marrow and (2) side effects of chemotherapy.

Cells in your bone marrow are constantly duplicating themselves to give rise to new blood cells. Just like any of the cells in your body, the cells in your bone marrow can also develop errors or mutations in their DNA as they are duplicating. If key mutations occur, this can lead to indefinite duplication of these cells. For example, if the cells responsible for making the white blood cells in your bone marrow start to duplicate indefinitely, without self-destructing, all of these new abnormal cells will be released into the bloodstream and cause an extreme elevation of the white blood cell count. This type of cancer is commonly referred to as *leukemia*, a cancer of the blood cells that starts in the bone marrow. Although the white blood cell count (the number of white blood cells measured in the blood with a blood test) is often very high in leukemia, the white blood cells are not functioning properly, and the person still has an increased susceptibility to infection. Eventually, because the abnormally dividing cells in the bone marrow can start to take over the limited space in the bone marrow, the production of normal cells ceases and the number of other blood cells in the blood decreases to abnormally low levels.

Think of a cookie factory. One day, for some unknown reason, an error develops in the wiring of the chocolate chip cookie machine and it starts to make abnormal chocolate chip cookies faster and faster, without shutting off. Some of these cookies have too many chocolate chips, some have none, some have too much butter, some not enough. Soon the entire factory is full of these abnormal chocolate chip cookies, and there is not room for the oatmeal raisin cookie machine or the peanut butter cookie machine to function normally. The trucks start to deliver the overproduced chocolate chip cookies to the stores, but these cookies are of no value to the store owners because they are abnormal in appearance and taste. Meanwhile, there is a shortage of oatmeal raisin and peanut butter cookies. Eventually, none of the trucks are able to deliver their cookies because the factory is in such disarray. Well, that is what happens to the bone marrow in leukemia.

Cancers that originate from cells in the bone marrow are often called "liquid" tumors, as opposed to cancers that start in solid organs such as the prostate, colon, breasts, lung, and so forth, which are called "solid" tumors. This is because the normal life of the blood cells is to circulate in the bloodstream; these cells are not normally confined to an organ. As a result, these

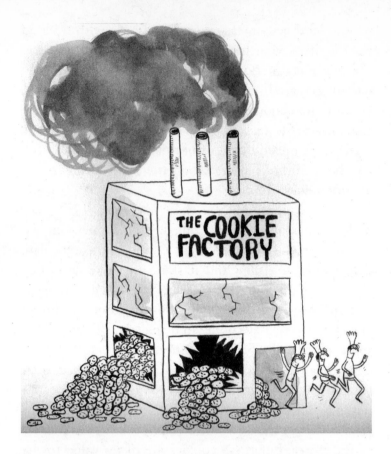

cancers are often detected by abnormal blood tests. In addition, we don't think of these cancers as localized or spreading (metastatic) in the same way that we do of cancers of solid organs. Liquid cancers tend to involve the bone marrow and the bloodstream and less commonly invade other organs. Because the abnormal cells that make up a liquid cancer are constantly circulating in the blood, these cancers are considered systemic from the get-go, and chemotherapy is often the primary treatment modality.

Another situation common in cancer that can cause the bone marrow to shut down, albeit temporarily, is receiving chemotherapy. In this case, the treatment of cancer, rather than the cancer itself, is at the root of the problem. Many chemotherapy drugs work by interfering with cells' ability to duplicate such that they are forced to die. The treatment is effective because cancer cells are generally the most rapidly dividing cells in the body. However, other cells in the body, such as the cells that produce the red blood cells, white blood cells, and platelets, can also be affected. As a result, about 10 to 14 days after receiving chemotherapy, the levels of these blood cells in the blood often decrease to abnormally low levels. The low amount of blood cells can be detected with a blood test. The bone marrow then recovers, starts making new cells, and the cells in the blood eventually return to normal levels. The impact of chemotherapy on the blood cells is discussed further in Chapter 9.

To make things a bit more complicated, your bone marrow makes different subsets of white blood cells. One of these subsets is called the *lymphocytes*. Once lymphocytes are released into the blood, they travel to your lymph nodes. Lymph nodes are small structures located throughout your body that are connected through an intricate network of vessels called *lymphatics*. You have about 600 lymph nodes in your body, with prominent areas in your neck, underarms, chest, and groin. You can think of the lymphatics as your body's sewer system and the lymph nodes as the waste stations. When you have an infection, the virus or bacterium that caused the infection is shuttled via the lymphatics to the lymph nodes where it can be destroyed by the lymphocytes. Remember when your mother used to check you for "swollen glands" by feeling your neck? These are not really glands—they are lymph nodes that become enlarged when your body is busy fighting off an infection.

Guess what? The lymphocytes in your lymph nodes can also duplicate, can also acquire errors resulting in indefinite duplication without self-destruction, and can thus form cancers. Cancers of the lymphocytes in lymph nodes are called *lymphomas*. Lymphomas fit somewhere in the middle of the schema of liquid and solid tumors. Lymphomas do involve blood cells; however, they often originate in a localized organ (in this case, a lymph node), and localized treatment (for example, radiation therapy) can sometimes play a role in addition to chemotherapy.

There is a common misconception that lymphoma is any cancer involving the lymph nodes. Rather, lymphoma is a cancer that starts in the lymphocytes, the cells

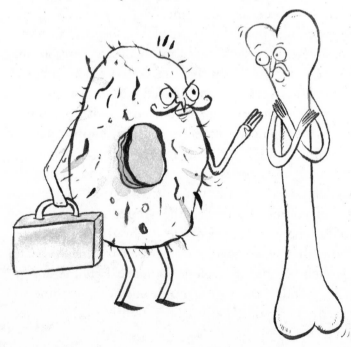

CALL ME BREAST CANCER.

that make up the lymph nodes. The behavior of cancers and, as a result, their treatment are determined by the cell type of origin. The lymph nodes are a very common first site of spread of various solid tumors. This makes sense because the lymphatic system is the sewer system that drains all of your organs. When cancer cells are growing and dividing, they can gain access to the lymphatics and spread to the lymph nodes. For example, when breast cancer spreads to the lymph nodes, it is called breast cancer that is metastatic to the lymph nodes, not lymphoma or lymph node cancer. This is an important distinction because these cancers are treated very differently. Similarly, when breast cancer spreads to the bone, this is called metastatic breast cancer to the bone rather than bone cancer; primary bone cancer is much less common and treated very differently.

CHAPTER 3

How is cancer diagnosed?

When there is a problem with your car, the problem might come to your attention in several different ways. The engine may make a funny sound, an alert light may illuminate on your dashboard, or the car may be slow to accelerate. The means by which the problem comes to your attention will differ depending on the specific location and details of the trouble as well as the age and make of the car. Most people will then bring the car to the repair shop where, in the age of advanced technology, the car is connected to a diagnostic machine to pinpoint the site of the problem. Although the diagnostic process is helpful, ultimately confirming the problem requires actually looking under the hood. At times, a part needs to be removed to determine the specifics of the problem. This is much like the process involved in diagnosing cancer.

Cancer presents (comes to the attention of a patient or physician) in many different ways. The symptoms or signs that lead to the detection of cancer depend on the type of cancer, the site of origin, and whether or not the cancer has spread. Sometimes, cancer is detected before there are symptoms present—think of the warning lights illuminating on the car dashboard. Because cancer involves an accumulation of cells growing uncontrollably, cancer can often be visualized

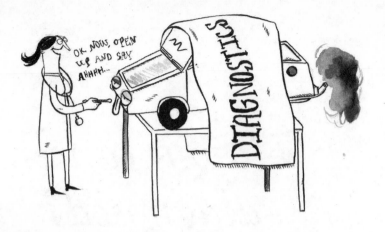

as a mass on an imaging test (for example, an X-ray or computed tomography [CT] scan). However, while blood tests and imaging tests can sometimes suggest a diagnosis of cancer, in almost all situations, with extremely rare exceptions, cancer must be diagnosed with a *biopsy*, a removal of a sample of tissue from the body. The reason a biopsy is necessary is because several other disorders such as an infectious or inflammatory process may mimic cancer on an imaging test. Remember, the diagnostic machine can be helpful in pinpointing the problem with your car, but to confirm the specifics of the problem usually requires "popping the hood."

Imaging tests generate pictures of your body or organs. Several different imaging tests can aid in the diagnosis of cancer and can help determine whether the cancer is localized or has spread. All of these tests provide pictures of the body; however, they often provide different and complementary information. Regardless of the type of imaging test, these scans are generally interpreted by a specialized physician called a *radiologist*. The radiologist looks at the pictures generated from the test, writes a report to describe the findings, and sends the report to the physician who ordered the test.

Once an abnormality is detected, typically a biopsy is performed. Again, a biopsy is a procedure used to obtain a sample of tissue from the body. The sample can be obtained in several different ways depending on the location of the abnormality in question. For example, if a mass can be felt on physical examination, such as an enlarged lymph node in the neck, a biopsy might be obtained by inserting a needle through the skin into the enlarged lymph node and aspirating (pulling out) tissue with a syringe. More commonly, abnormalities that are deep within the body are detected by imaging tests. In the past, a surgical procedure in the operating room (with the patient under anesthesia) was required to obtain a tissue sample of the internal organs or other tissues deep within the body. These days, biopsies of masses deep within the body often can be performed under radiographic guidance. That is, a radiologist can detect the location of the abnormality on an imaging test, such as a CT scan, and then take pictures while he or she inserts a needle through the skin to be sure that the needle is entering the area of abnormality. The tissue is then withdrawn through a hollow needle. The procedure is done with the patient awake, although sedative medicines are usually given and numbing medicine is used to minimize pain from insertion of the needle.

Other common types of biopsies involved in diagnosing cancer include endoscopic biopsies (biopsies taken by visualizing an abnormality with a thin flexible scope, often performed for abnormalities in the colon, stomach, or lungs) and bone marrow biopsies (biopsies using a hollow needle inserted into the back of the pelvic bone to examine the bone marrow, the "factory" of the blood cells).

After the sample is obtained, the tissue is processed to allow the cells to be viewed under a microscope. Remember, these cells are incredibly small and as a result, require a microscope at very high magnification to visualize. The biopsy specimen is then viewed by a pathologist, a doctor with special training in interpreting biopsy tissue. The pathologist is able to look at the tissue under the microscope and make a diagnosis based on the appearance of the cells. Because cancer cells are damaged or abnormal cells, they look different from normal cells. A pathologist can determine whether there is evidence of cancer in a biopsy specimen and can also generally determine what type of cancer is present. For example, if cancerous, a mass in the lung could represent a cancer that started in the lung or could represent cancer cells that started in another organ and spread to the lung. Even cancers that start in a particular organ can come in different "flavors." Lung cancers are often called small cell cancer or non-small cell cancer based on the appearance of the cells under the microscope. This is a critical distinction because small cell and non-small cell lung cancers are treated differently.

Pathologists can often get a sense for how aggressive cancer cells look under the microscope, called the *grade* of the cancer. The aggressiveness of the cells tells the doctor a bit about the chance that these cells will spread to other places in the body.

Newer techniques have greatly expanded the type of information that can be learned from a biopsy specimen. As discussed in Chapter 1, cancer results from damage to DNA that allows cells to grow uncontrollably without dying. As these cells are growing and dividing, additional damage to DNA typically occurs, often contributing to the ability of the cancer cells to grow and spread. Remember, DNA is the instruction manual that your cells use to make proteins. Damaged DNA results in damaged proteins. These proteins can often be measured by pathologists using special types of stains. Measuring these proteins can be important for two reasons. First, an elevated (or decreased) level of a certain protein may provide additional information about the cancer cells' aggressiveness and ability to spread. Second, and perhaps more important, the presence of a certain protein informs the doctor that a certain treatment may be particularly effective. For instance, pathologists routinely analyze breast cancer specimens for the presence of an increased amount of a protein called Her-2. The presence of an increased amount of this protein indicates that the drug trastuzumab may be an effective treatment. Trastuzumab is useful because increased amounts of Her-2 can promote the growth and spread of breast cancer, and trastuzumab blocks this action of Her-2. An intense area of research is attempting to identify similar tests and treatments for other types of cancers.

CHAPTER 4

What is a pathology report?

As noted in Chapter 3, a diagnosis of cancer is ultimately made by a pathologist reviewing a sample of tissue under a microscope. After reviewing the tissue, the pathologist generates a pathology report describing the findings. This report often contains key information about the cancer, including indicators of prognosis and indicators of which treatments might be most effective. Therefore, it is useful to understand how to read a pathology report. **Table 4-1** is a sample pathology report from a patient who underwent surgery for breast cancer.

The amount of data contained on a pathology report depends on the source of the tissue. A needle biopsy consists of a very small fragment of tissue, and the report may consist of only one line describing the type of cancer. For example, if a patient has a solitary lung mass and multiple liver masses on a computed tomography (CT) scan, a situation suspicious for lung cancer that has spread to the liver, a needle biopsy of a liver mass might be performed to confirm the diagnosis. A pathology report in this situation might state, "malignant cells, consistent with metastatic small cell lung cancer." A pathology report from a surgery to remove cancer from the body along with the

Table 4-1 Sample Pathology Report

ANATOMIC PATHOLOGY REPORT

PATIENT: SMITH, JANE
D.O.B.: 5/12/1942
SPECIMEN #: SZ:S11-3402
PHYSICIAN: DR. JONES

CLINICAL HISTORY: BREAST CANCER
SPECIMEN(S):
    A. RIGHT AXILLARY SENTINEL LYMPH NODE #1
    B. RIGHT AXILLARY SENTINEL LYMPH NODE #2
    C. RIGHT LUMPECTOMY

FINAL DIAGNOSIS

    A. SENTINEL LYMPH NODE #1, RIGHT AXILLARY, BIOPSY:
        NO TUMOR IDENTIFIED IN ONE LYMPH NODE (0/1)

    B. SENTINEL LYMPH NODE #2, RIGHT AXILLARY, BIOPSY:
        NO TUMOR IDENTIFIED IN ONE LYMPH NODE (0/1)

    C. RIGHT BREAST, LUMPECTOMY:
        INFILTRATING DUCTAL CARCINOMA
        Tumor location: UPPER OUTER QUADRANT
        Size of invasive tumor: 2.2 x 0.9 x 0.7 CM.
        Nottingham histology grade: 3 OF 3, POORLY DIFFERENTIATED.
        Lymphatic/vascular invasion: NOT IDENTIFIED
        Surgical margins: NEGATIVE BY AT LEAST 1 CM

ADDENDUM*

BREAST PROGNOSTIC STUDIES

ESTROGEN RECEPTOR (ER):	4%
PROGRESTERONE RECEPTOR (PR):	0%
PROLIFERATION RATE (Ki67):	31%
HER2/NEU:	STRONGLY POSITIVE (3+)

---

lymph nodes located near the cancer (like the report in Table 4-1) typically contains much more information.

The first bit of information that you should look for on the pathology report is the *histology*, essentially a description of what the cells look like under the microscope. Typically, the cancers that arise in specific organs have a common histology. For example, the sample pathology report indicates that the breast cancer is an infiltrating ductal carcinoma. The other most common histology of breast cancer is called lobular carcinoma. The histology is of significance because it conveys information about the behavior of the can-

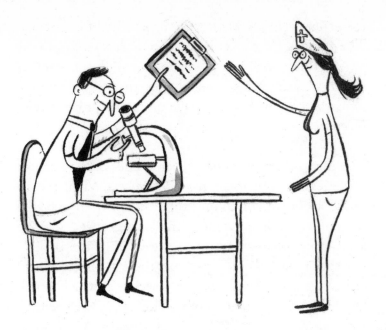

cer and may dictate the appropriate treatment. For instance, small cell cancer of the lung is almost never treated with surgery, whereas non-small cell cancer of the lung is treated with surgery if the cancer has not spread beyond the lung.

The *grade* of the cancer refers to how aggressive or immature the cells appear under the microscope. Depending on the type of cancer, the grade may be designated with a number (such as grades 1–4) or by a description (for example, low grade, high grade). Another way of stating this information is to describe the cells as well differentiated, moderately differentiated, or poorly differentiated. Well-differentiated cancers, or low-grade cancers, appear more like normal cells and, therefore, commonly grow more slowly and behave less aggressively. Poorly differentiated cancers, or high-grade cancers, generally grow faster and behave more aggressively. You can see in the sample pathology report that the cancer is grade 3 out of 3, or poorly differentiated. The grade of the cancer is completely different from the *stage* of the cancer. The grade does not indicate whether or not a cancer has spread, as does the stage, although higher grade cancers may have more of a propensity to spread.

The *margin* status of the cancer applies only to cancer surgeries and not to biopsy specimens. When a cancer or an organ containing the cancer is removed, the surgeon attempts to remove the entire cancer. If there are cancer cells extending to the edge of the pathology specimen, this indicates that there are likely cancer cells on the other edge of that specimen, which is still located in the patient's body. This is called a *positive margin*.

Think about a raisin in a loaf of bread. Now imagine trying to cut the loaf of bread so that the entire raisin is contained in the half of the loaf that is closest to you. Pick up that half of the loaf and look at the side of the bread where your knife cut the loaf in half. If you can see the raisin all the way up to the edge of that side, chances are there is still part of the raisin in the other half of the loaf sitting on the table (you can probably even see a small piece of the raisin in that half). This raisin extending all the way to the edge of your bread "specimen" is the equivalent of a positive margin. On the other hand, if the raisin is embedded deep in the half of the bread that you removed, then you "got it all"; this is the equivalent of a *negative margin*.

Pathology reports may state that the margins were negative, indicating that there was normal tissue between the cancer and the edge of the specimen, or the report might describe the distance between the cancer cells and the edge of the specimen (for example, the margins were negative by 1 cm). Clearly, the goal of a cancer surgery is to have negative margins. However, if the margins are positive, this information may guide further treatment after surgery. In the sample pathology report, the margins are negative by at least 1 cm, meaning that there is at least 1 cm of normal tissue between cancer cells and any of the edges of the surgical specimen.

When a surgeon says he or she "got it all," this typically refers to the fact that the cancer was removed completely with negative margins. Achieving negative margins indicates that there is unlikely to be any cancer cells left behind in the region where the cancer was removed. Unfortunately, achieving negative margins does not necessarily ensure that microscopic cancer cells did not spread to other areas of the body before surgery (see Chapter 5).

The status of the regional lymph nodes, the lymph nodes nearest the organ where the cancer originated, is usually included in pathology reports from cancer surgeries. Most pathology reports describe the number of lymph nodes removed, in addition to the number of lymph nodes involved with cancer. Whether or not the lymph nodes are involved with cancer is of major prognostic importance. Also, if the lymph nodes are involved with cancer, this may suggest the need for additional treatment. In the sample pathology report, there were two lymph nodes described (specimens A and B), neither of which was involved with cancer.

For many cancers, the pathologist will look for the level of expression of certain proteins by staining the biopsy specimen with special stains. As described in Chapter 3, these proteins may convey information about prognosis, or these proteins may suggest which treatments might be most effective for a particular cancer. At the bottom of the sample pathology report, the presence (and amount) of certain proteins relevant to prognosis and treatment of breast cancer are shown. Each different type of cancer is associated with different proteins of importance. For some cancers, proteins that are important with regard to treatment and prognosis have not yet been identified, and as a result, this section will be absent from the pathology report.

Pathology reports for "liquid" tumors often involve a lymph node biopsy or a bone marrow biopsy. The information contained in reports of these types of biopsies is somewhat different from what is previously described. Because there are so many different types of leukemias and lymphomas, a combination of the appearance of the cancer cells under the microscope (histology) and the presence of certain proteins on the cells analyzed with a technique called *flow cytometry* is often used to make the specific diagnosis. With some liquid cancers, all patients have the same specific gene mutation (error in the instruction manual) that leads to the development of the cancer. For example, patients with chronic myeloid leukemia have a mutation that leads to joining of two genes together (*bcr-abl*) that normally are not located near one another in the DNA—think about the pages in the instruction manual being stuck together. This results in an abnormal signal telling the white blood cells to divide continuously. This abnormal gene can be tested for in the blood or bone marrow and is used to make the diagnosis of chronic myeloid leukemia.

CHAPTER 5

What is cancer "staging"? How is cancer treated?

Have you ever seen footage on the evening news of a blazing California forest fire? Typically, there is a shot of a small airplane flying overhead dousing the flames below. Well, a forest fire is perhaps one of the best ways to think about the different stages of cancer and the different treatment options available.

Like cancer, forest fires start as a localized event. One tree in a vast forest might catch fire. Like cancer, over time, the fire may start to spread. The single tree that started the fire spreads some flames to the next tree, which then ignites the next tree, and so on. When flying overhead and viewing a small cluster of trees ablaze, a forest fire might appear localized. With cancer, *staging* examinations are performed to determine whether a cancer is localized or whether the cancer has spread. Generally, staging examinations involve one or more imaging tests: computed tomography (CT) scans, magnetic resonance imaging (MRI) scans, bone scans, and positron emission tomography (PET) scans. When these imaging tests reveal no evidence of spread, then the cancer is considered localized.

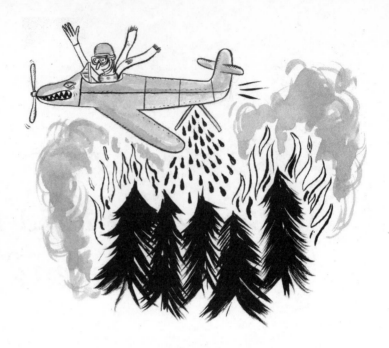

If a single tree is on fire, and there has been no spread of the fire to the rest of the forest, then concentrating all efforts on that single tree is typically the best approach to stop the fire. Similarly, when there is no evidence that a cancer has spread, local treatment approaches are generally utilized. There are two major *local* treatment options for cancer. Surgery can remove the cancer or the organ in which the cancer arose. Alternatively, radiation therapy can be directed at the cancer in an attempt to kill the cancer cells. Think of radiation therapy like a flashlight: it is a beam that can be aimed at a specific location in the body to kill cells in that location. Localized treatments (surgery or radiation) for cancers that have not spread are often curative.

When there is evidence that a forest fire is raging throughout the forest, then concentrating all of the efforts on the tree that started the fire does little to address the problem at hand. Rather, a solution is needed to control the entire fire, such as sending out planes to spray the whole forest. Frequently, when patients have a cancer that has spread from one part of the body to other organs (metastatic cancer), questions arise about the need for surgery to remove the organ from which the cancer arose. Considering the forest fire analogy, it becomes clear that removing the prostate of a man with prostate cancer that has spread to the bones would do little to address the bigger problem—that the cancer has already spread. Rather, a *systemic* treatment is needed. Chemotherapy is the major systemic treatment used to treat cancer. *Chemotherapy* refers to medication that can potentially kill cancer cells. Chemotherapy is a systemic treatment because the medications circulate in the bloodstream and can reach cancer cells wherever they might be located in the body. When cancer has spread to distant parts of the body, chemotherapy can be an effective means of shrinking the cancer, improving cancer-related symptoms, delaying spread of the cancer, and ultimately prolonging life. However, for most cancers of solid organs (with some exceptions), this treatment is generally not curative when cancer has spread to other organs or distant locations in the body. Consider the forest fire—the plane may not be able to extinguish the entire fire if some parts of the forest are difficult to reach. However, the pilot may still be successful in delaying the spread of the fire and limiting the damage from the fire. There are still several reasons to "treat" the fire even if ultimately the fire cannot be completely eradicated.

You may have heard of someone who had cancer treated with a local therapy (surgery or radiation) and the cancer "came back" in a distant organ years later. How does this happen? Well, the cancer didn't really come back—it never left in the first place. What do I mean by this? When staging examinations are performed when a cancer is diagnosed, the ability to detect spread of the cancer is somewhat limited by the technology of current imaging tests. Even with the most advanced technology available, imaging tests can generally detect only cancer cells that have accumulated to form a mass approximately 1 cm in size. It takes approximately 1,000,000,000 cancer cells to form a mass 1 cm in size! Clearly, the spread of 1,000 or even 1,000,000 cancer cells is easily missed with the current technology. The term for these cancer cells that have spread but that are too small to be seen with current imaging tests is *micrometastases* (in other words, microscopic metastases). Over time, however, these cells can continue to grow and divide to the point where they can be visualized on a scan. At that point, the "recurrence" is detected.

Think again of the forest fire. A plane is sent out to survey the fire and it appears that only a single tree is on fire. Therefore, this single tree is doused with water until the fire is out. Now from up in the air, no other areas appear to be on fire. However, from that vantage point, it is easy to miss the few sparks that had spread from tree to tree and that are slowly gaining in intensity (like micrometastases). If, from the air, no other evidence of fire could be detected, but there is a strong suspicion that the fire might have spread because of the conditions (perhaps a very windy day), it might make sense to spray the remainder of the forest to squelch any sparks before they become problematic. Well, this situation is analogous to the use of adjuvant chemotherapy in cancer. *Adjuvant chemotherapy* refers to treatment given after (or before) surgery or radiation for localized cancer to kill microscopic cells that might have spread. The rationale for this approach is that microscopic cancer cells that have spread may be killed with chemotherapy and result in a cure of the cancer that would not have been achieved with surgery alone.

Commonly, there is no evidence of distant spread of a cancer when the initial staging imaging tests are performed, but there are features of the cancer that suggest that the patient is at very high risk for having these micrometastases. Consider a patient with breast cancer who has the tumor in her breast removed, a procedure often referred to as a *lumpectomy*. Some lymph nodes in the underarm are generally removed as well because these lymph nodes are typically the first site of potential spread of breast cancer cells. When examined under the microscope, there may be evidence of cancer cells in the lymph nodes (by definition, these are micrometastases because these cells could only be visualized under the microscope). These micrometastases to the lymph node are not a problem because they are in the pathology lab and no longer in the patient's body. However, it is the implication of this microscopic cancer in the lymph nodes that is of concern. The presence of these micrometastases in the lymph nodes suggests a high risk for microscopic cancer cells spread to other sites in the body as well, despite imaging tests showing no evidence of spread. As a result, chemotherapy is given after surgery in an attempt to kill these microscopic cancer cells. Again, this is called *adjuvant* chemotherapy because the treatment is given as an adjuvant to some form of local treatment (such as surgery or radiation).

Back to the forest fire. Because small sparks cannot be seen from the airplane, it is not clear whether some other trees have an early fire brewing. The whole forest is sprayed "just in case," and only in time will it become apparent whether the entire fire has been extinguished. The same is true of each patient treated with adjuvant chemotherapy after surgery. In any individual patient, it is not known whether distant micrometastases are present. Currently, no test available can detect *microscopic* spread of cancer to other organs in the body—this would require removal of every organ and examination of each one under the microscope. Therefore, if chemotherapy is administered after the lumpectomy, and 5 years later there is no evidence of cancer, it is not clear whether the chemotherapy killed the micrometastases or whether they were never present in the first place. To determine whether such treatments are beneficial, randomized clinical trials have been performed. For example, thousands of women with localized breast cancer who were thought to be at high risk for microscopic spread of their cancer (based on features of the primary tumor under the microscope) have been randomized in clinical trials to surgery alone or surgery followed by chemotherapy. In general, these studies have shown that years later, more women were alive who received the surgery plus chemotherapy compared with women treated with surgery alone, proving that the addition of chemotherapy cured some patients who would not have been cured with surgery alone. Only through these scientific studies has the benefit of adjuvant chemotherapy been proven, and this approach is now routinely employed in a variety of cancers including breast cancer, colon cancer, lung cancer, and ovarian cancer.

Staging simply refers to testing performed to determine where the cancer is and where it is not. The most common staging system used in solid tumors involves the TNM classification, which refers to the status of the primary tumor (T), whether the lymph nodes near the primary tumor are involved (N), and whether or not there has been distant spread of the cancer (M). These groupings are then compiled to assign the cancer to a stage from I to IV. However, as can be gleaned from the preceding discussion, these precise staging details are probably not as relevant to the patient as whether the cancer is localized, is localized but thought to be at high risk for microscopic spread (sometimes called locally advanced), or has spread (metastatic). These are the distinctions that ultimately guide the treatment of solid tumors, as shown in **Table 5-1**.

Staging was initially developed so that doctors could compare notes to determine the prognosis of patients with similar types of cancers and to determine which treatments were most beneficial. Staging is meant to be static. The stage of a cancer is assigned at the time of diagnosis. However, cancer is often not static and the extent of the cancer, prognosis, and treatment may change during the course of a patient's illness. For example, a patient may be diagnosed with breast cancer that has spread to the lymph nodes in the underarm after undergoing surgery to remove the cancer. This diagnosis is referred to as locally advanced breast cancer,

Table 5-1 Stages of Cancer and Their Treatment

Status of Cancer	Treatment
Localized	• Surgery or radiation
Localized but high risk for microscopic spread (also known as locally advanced)	• Surgery +/– adjuvant chemotherapy • Radiation +/– adjuvant or concurrent chemotherapy
Spread (also known as metastatic)	• Chemotherapy • Radiation therapy or surgery may still be used to treat symptoms (e.g., radiation therapy to the bone from a site of cancer causing pain)

or stage II or III breast cancer, depending on the details of the size of the cancer and the number of lymph nodes involved. A CT scan and PET scan reveal no evidence of spread of the cancer to distant sites in the body, and the patient is then treated with approximately 4 months of adjuvant chemotherapy after surgery. Many patients are cured with this approach and will never require further treatment. Unfortunately, 2 years later, the patient in the example develops evidence of cancer in the lungs and liver on a CT scan. A biopsy of a liver mass is performed and confirms that this is breast cancer that has spread to the liver. The adjuvant chemotherapy in this example was unsuccessful in killing the microscopic cells that spread to the lungs and liver even before the cancer was removed. The cancer is now termed metastatic because there is evidence of cancer in other organs that can be seen on the scans. The specific treatment regimen, prognosis, and goals of treatment have also changed because the cancer is no longer considered *localized with a high risk for spread* but now is considered *spread* or *metastatic*.

It is a somewhat confusing concept that chemotherapy given in the adjuvant setting (after surgery or radiation) can be potentially curative whereas chemotherapy given when cancer has definitively spread is generally not curative. Whether the chemotherapy can be curative has to do with the volume or number of cancer cells that have spread. When small numbers of cancer cells have spread in a microscopic fashion, chemotherapy can potentially wipe out all of those cancer cells and result in a cure of the cancer. All of the cancer cells must be killed because even one remaining cancer cell can continue to grow and divide and cause a recurrence of the cancer. When cancer cells have clearly spread to others sites in the body, the number of cancer cells in the body can be billions of times more than in the micrometastatic situation. It is much more difficult for chemotherapy to kill this large volume of cancer cells, and that is why the treatment can be effective but is generally not curative. I stress *generally* because there are cancers that have spread to other organs that are commonly cured, such as metastatic testicular cancer. In addition, a very small subset of patients with a variety of metastatic solid tumors (for example, bladder cancer) may be cured with chemotherapy (along with other treatments including surgery). The reason why some individuals' cancers are so sensitive to killing by chemotherapy and others' are not is not clear, but is an area of intense research.

Another form of combined modality treatment commonly used in the treatment of cancer is the use of radiation and chemotherapy at the same time. This is called concurrent *chemoradiation*. Giving chemotherapy at the same time as radiation can enhance the effectiveness of radiation. A common cancer where this type of treatment is used is cancer of the larynx (voice box). In the past, treatment of larynx cancer required removing the voice box, leaving patients unable to speak. Now, larynx cancer is often treated with the combination of chemotherapy and radiation given at the same time. This treatment can lead to curing the cancer while sparing patients from an operation to remove their voice box.

I should note that the discussions in this chapter generally refer to the management of solid tumors. Liquid cancers (for example, leukemias), because they involve blood or bone marrow, are generally considered systemic from the outset, and chemotherapy is typically a major component of treatment and sometimes the only treatment modality utilized. Many liquid cancers, including certain leukemias and lymphomas, are very sensitive to chemotherapy and are potentially curable despite involving the bone marrow, blood, and sometimes lymph nodes in many different locations in the body.

CHAPTER 6

Why do I have to see more than one kind of doctor?

Cancer is a multidisciplinary disease. That is, managing cancer typically requires the expertise of several different types of physicians. The involvement of these different physicians depends somewhat on the type and stage of the cancer.

Primary care physicians are often involved in the diagnosis of cancer. Primary care physicians, typically internists or family practitioners, have spent 3 years of training after medical school (called a residency) to become proficient in the skills required to practice general medicine. Many patients initially seek consultation with their primary physician for evaluation of new or concerning symptoms or may have abnormal findings detected at the time of a routine physical. Often, primary care physicians order the blood work, or imaging tests, that lead to the suspicion of a cancer diagnosis. Alternatively, the primary care physician may have recommended the screening mammogram or colonoscopy that led to the detection of cancer. Depending on the primary care physician and the relationship a

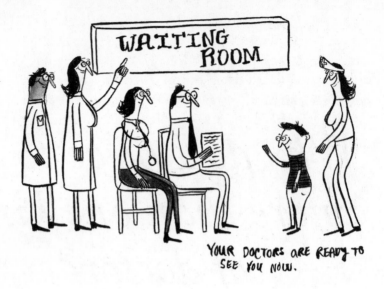

YOUR DOCTORS ARE READY TO SEE YOU NOW.

patient has fostered with him or her, this physician may also play an integral role during the treatment of cancer.

Medical oncologists are doctors who have completed a 3-year residency in internal medicine after medical school and then decided to subspecialize in the management of patients with cancer. To subspecialize, an additional 2 to 3 years of training, called a fellowship, is required. Medical oncologists are also sometimes called chemotherapy doctors because chemotherapy is the major treatment modality used by them. Most medical oncologists are also trained in hematology, the study and treatment of diseases of the blood.

Radiation oncologists, as the name implies, are doctors who are trained in the use of radiation therapy for the treatment of cancer. Radiation oncologists complete 1 year of general medical training after medical school, called an internship, and then complete a 4-year residency in radiation oncology.

Surgeons may be involved with the initial diagnosis of cancer, may perform potentially curative surgery for cancer, and may perform surgeries to alleviate symptoms related to advanced cancer. General surgeons are surgeons with broad general training in surgery and, in addition to performing cancer operations, commonly perform other operations as well (such as appendix surgery hernia repairs). General surgeons complete 5 years of training in surgery (general surgery residency) after graduating medical school. These surgeons are commonly involved with cancer operations of the breast and gastrointestinal tract (including the stomach, small intestine, or colon). Other surgical subspecialists focus on particular areas of the body and commonly perform cancer operations. These surgeons generally spend 1 to 2 years after medical school training in general surgery, and then complete residency programs focusing on a particular area of the body. Head and neck surgeons (also called otolaryngologists) are involved with surgery for cancers of the mouth, throat, and voice box. Thoracic surgeons perform surgery for lung cancers. For most of these surgical specialties, fellowship programs are available that provide additional training focused on cancer surgeries, and surgeons completing this advanced training are often referred to as surgical oncologists.

Nurses and midlevel practitioners (physician assistants and nurse practitioners) in each of the disciplines described previously play key roles in the care of patients with cancer. These individuals often have the most regular contact with patients, are experts in managing the side effects of cancer therapies, and provide support and counseling. Chemotherapy nurses are experts in the administration of chemotherapy, which requires a vast array of knowledge because each chemotherapy medication has a specific method of administration.

The pathologist and radiologist are two of the most important physicians involved in the care of the cancer patient, but patients rarely meet these physicians because these specialists generally work behind the scenes. The pathologist's role is critical because interpreting a biopsy or surgical specimen and making the proper diagnosis are essential to selecting the appropriate treatment. Pathologists complete a 4-year residency in pathology after medical school. When imaging studies (such as CT scans and bone scans) are performed, a physician is needed to look at the images and interpret them. That physician is a radiologist. Radiologists are crucial not only in determining whether a patient might have cancer but also in determining whether the cancer is localized or has spread. These physicians are also involved in determining whether patients are responding to treatment by comparing the results of a scan prior to treatment with a scan after treatment. Radiologists complete 1 year of general medical training after graduating medical school, followed by 4 years of training in radiology.

Interventional radiologists are playing a larger role in the care of patients with cancer. These are radiologists who specialize in performing minimally invasive procedures under radiographic guidance. In lay terms, that means that while the radiologist is looking at an image of a patient's insides, he or she inserts small needles through the skin (after giving numbing medication and typically after patients have received sedative medications) to take tissue samples from an area of abnormality. This is called a radiographic-guided biopsy. With increasing frequency, this is the procedure that leads to the initial diagnosis of cancer. Interventional radiologists are also developing new ways to treat specific areas of cancer in the body by manipulating needles or catheters (small tubes) while visualizing an image of patients' insides and applying a treatment to the site of abnormalities with this approach. For instance, an interventional radiologist may insert a probe into a liver tumor and freeze the tumor or burn the tumor using techniques called cryoablation or radiofrequency ablation, respectively. Interventional radiologists generally spend a year of additional training in interventional procedures (fellowship) after completing radiology residency.

CHAPTER 7

What is chemotherapy?

The reasons why chemotherapy might be recommended for the treatment of cancer are discussed in Chapter 5. These reasons for solid tumors are as follows:

- Treatment given as an adjuvant to local treatments (such as surgery or radiation) in an attempt to kill microscopic cancer cells that might have spread throughout the body
- Treatment given at the same time as radiation to enhance the effectiveness of radiation
- Treatment given as a primary therapy for metastatic cancer

For liquid tumors, chemotherapy is often the mainstay of treatment because these cancers travel in the blood and are considered systemic from the outset.

Chemotherapy is a general term used for medications that can potentially kill cancer cells. More than 100 different chemotherapy medications are commonly used to treat cancer, and the list is growing as new drugs are developed and approved for use by the Food and Drug Administration. *Cytotoxic chemotherapy* is the term used for the traditional chemotherapy drugs that work by interfering with

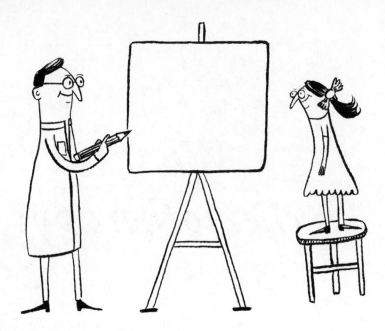

cells' ability to duplicate their genetic material (instruction manual). Because all of your cells have genetic material that needs to be copied for the cells to duplicate, cytotoxic chemotherapy is relatively selective for cancer cells only because these cells are more rapidly growing than other cells in the body are. Killing other rapidly dividing cells in the body may cause many of the common side effects associated with chemotherapy. For example, hair loss may occur because the cells responsible for hair growth are killed, and nausea, vomiting, and diarrhea can occur because the cells lining the intestines are killed.

A newer class of drugs developed to attack cancer is generally referred to as *targeted therapy*. Many of these drugs try to block a particular protein or cell function present only in cancer cells, thereby sparing normal cells and limiting the side effects of treatment. When targeted drugs were initially being developed, they were often referred to as *magic bullets* because of the proposed specificity for cancer cells. In reality, the targets of most of these drugs are also found on some normal cells in the body, and like traditional cytotoxic chemotherapy, these drugs are also associated with potential side effects. The side effects from these newer drugs, however, tend to be quite different from side effects of traditional chemotherapy and are dependent on the target of the medications. Some side effects of these newer drugs may include an acne-like rash, diarrhea, sores on the hands and toes, or high blood pressure. Many modern chemotherapy regimens involve a targeted drug given in combination with a traditional chemotherapy drug.

Instead of attempting to block a specific protein in a cancer cell, some targeted therapies block a mechanism in the body that the cancer cell hijacks and then uses to its advantage to grow. Like normal cells, cancer cells need oxygen and nutrients to grow. Cells rely on blood vessels to bring them oxygen and nutrients. Cancer cells can send signals to blood vessels to sprout new vessels to feed tumors; this is called *angiogenesis*. Antiangiogenic drugs are available to block this new blood vessel formation with the goal of starving cancer cells. These drugs have been incorporated into the standard treatment of many cancers.

Some cancers are fueled by normal hormones that exist in the body. For example, estrogen can cause certain breast cancers to grow, and testosterone can cause prostate cancers to grow. Treatments to block these hormones, often called hormonal therapy (although probably better referred to as anti-hormonal therapy), play a key role in the treatment of these cancers. These hormonal therapies are typically given as pills or injections, and the side effects mainly result from loss of the natural hormones in the body. Decreasing the level of testosterone in men treated for prostate cancer can cause hot flashes, loss of muscle mass, and difficulty achieving erections, and using estrogen-blocking drugs in women can cause hot flashes, vaginal dryness, and loss of libido.

Some chemotherapy medications are administered intravenously whereas others are administered orally. These days, when chemotherapy medications are given intravenously, they can typically be given in the oncologist's office rather than requiring admission to a hospital. Each time the chemotherapy is administered, an intravenous line (IV) is placed. Alternatively, patients may have a port placed. The port is a small device that is inserted under the skin (either by an interventional radiologist or surgeon) in the upper chest wall or the forearm. The port looks like a nickel-sized protrusion in the skin. The device has a spongy diaphragm in the center that can be accessed by placing a small needle through the skin. This allows access to the vein in which the port is inserted, and the chemotherapy can then be infused through this port for each treatment without having a new IV placed in a different vein for each chemotherapy session.

Because there are so many chemotherapy drugs, the type of chemotherapy regimen that a patient receives is selected by the medical oncologist based on the type of cancer, with consideration given to the patient's prior treatment, organ function, and other medical problems. Sometimes a single chemotherapy medicine is appropriate, and other times a regimen combining several medications is appropriate. The recommendations are based on which chemotherapy regimens have proved to be beneficial for a particular type of cancer in clinical trials that have been performed in the past; drugs are not just chosen at random. For example, a clinical trial might have shown that chemotherapy X works better than does chemotherapy Y for breast cancer. Then, chemotherapy X becomes a new standard treatment for breast cancer. Often, several "standard" regimens are acceptable for each cancer, and therefore, recommendations may differ from one doctor to another. In some cases, the choice of chemotherapy drugs is tailored according to specific proteins expressed by the cancer, which the pathologist can test for during analysis of the tumor. For instance, breast cancer cells may have hormone receptors (for example, the estrogen receptor), a protein called Her-2, or neither of these proteins. Which receptors are found in the cells directly influences the choice of treatment because these proteins predict which treatments might work the best.

Each chemotherapy medication is given at a specific dose and schedule as determined based on early studies with the particular drug. The dose is most often individualized to a patient and is commonly based on a formula known as the body surface area, or BSA. This formula takes into account a patient's height and weight. Some chemotherapy medication dosages are based on kidney function, weight alone, or are a fixed dose for all patients.

Several individuals are involved in the administration of chemotherapy. The oncologist orders the medications and calculates the appropriate doses. A pharmacist mixes the chemotherapy in the appropriate solution and prepares the bags labeled with the patient's name and dose to be administered. A chemotherapy nurse either places an IV or accesses a patient's port and then infuses the chemotherapy medication over the appropriate amount of time. The length of time it takes to administer a chemotherapy medication depends on the particular medication. Some medications are administered by IV push. This means that the nurse takes a syringe prepared with the chemotherapy and pushes the medication into the IV or port over a period of minutes. Other chemotherapy medications are infused (meaning that bags of the chemotherapy are slowly dripped into the IV or port through long tubing) over periods of time ranging from less than an hour to several hours. The chemotherapy infusion should be painless, and there are generally no immediate symptoms while the chemotherapy is being infused, although sometimes nausea or allergic reactions can occur. Chemotherapy nurses are always nearby during treatment in case of these reactions.

Chemotherapy is typically given in *cycles*. This is just a way for the oncologist to keep track of how many treatments have been given. A cycle may last 1 week, 2 weeks, 4 weeks, or longer, depending on the particular regimen. When chemotherapy regimens involve multiple drugs, the individual drugs may be given on different days during the cycle. Consider the following example of the four-drug MVAC regimen used to treat bladder cancer. (MVAC stands for the first letter of each drug name used in the treatment.) A cycle of MVAC lasts 28 days, but the individual drugs are administered on specific days during the cycle as follows:

Methotrexate on days 1, 15, and 22

Vinblastine on days 2, 15, and 22

Adriamycin on day 2

Cisplatin on day 2

The number of cycles of chemotherapy that each patient requires depends on the type of cancer, the length of the cycle, and the circumstance in which chemotherapy is being administered. When there has been no identifiable spread of cancer on scans and the treatment is being administered as adjuvant chemotherapy after surgery or radiation, treatment is often given for 4 to 6 months. When cancer has already spread (metastasized) on scans, chemotherapy is often given for 2 to 3 months, and then the scans are repeated to determine whether the treatment is working. Treatment is then continued for another fixed duration of time, and the scans are repeated, and so on.

The first chemotherapy regimen used to treat a patient with cancer that has spread to other parts of the body is often referred to as first-line chemotherapy. The response of a patient with metastatic cancer to a particular chemotherapy regimen generally falls into one of four categories:

- A complete response (also sometimes referred to as a complete remission) refers to a situation when the cancer can no longer be seen on follow-up scans.
- A partial response means that the cancer has decreased in size but is still visible on a scan.
- Stable disease is just like it sounds—the cancer has neither grown nor shrunk on follow-up scans.
- Progressive disease means that the cancer continues to grow despite the chemotherapy.

When a response (complete or partial) or stable disease is achieved with chemotherapy, the chemotherapy is either continued for a fixed duration of time (for example, 6 months) or continued until the cancer begins to grow again. This depends somewhat on the type of the cancer and somewhat on the practice of the particular oncologist. If follow-up scans reveal progression of the cancer, then another chemotherapy regimen is often utilized. This is referred to as second-line chemotherapy. Different drugs are then used because the cancer cells are resistant to the prior chemotherapy regimen. Many patients go on to receive additional "lines" of chemotherapy (for example, third-line chemotherapy, fourth-line chemotherapy) with new regimens being initiated when the prior regimen no longer controls the cancer. In this manner, some cancers can be managed for a prolonged period of time with ongoing treatments much in the way other chronic diseases are managed.

Remember, the response categories described earlier really refer to patients receiving chemotherapy for metastatic cancer. When patients are receiving chemotherapy after surgery in the adjuvant setting, there is by definition no evidence of metastatic cancer on scans prior to starting chemotherapy. The response to chemotherapy is difficult to assess in this setting and really is determined only by the test of time—if the cancer never recurs, then either the chemotherapy worked and killed all of the microscopic cancer cells that had spread or there was no microscopic spread of the cancer in the first place. If the cancer appears in a distant site in the body at some later time, this is called a recurrence (really a misnomer as described in Chapter 5) and treatment generally involves a different chemotherapy regimen than the regimen used in the adjuvant setting.

The effectiveness of chemotherapy is dependent on the situation in which the chemotherapy is being administered, the type of cancer, and whether or not the patient has received prior treatment. Perhaps most important, the effectiveness of chemotherapy is dependent on the biology of an individual's cancer—cancer originating in the same organ and spreading to the same location in two different individuals might respond very differently to the same chemotherapy. For one patient, the cancer may completely disappear on the follow-up scan whereas in the other patient, there may be further growth and spread of the cancer. Researchers are learning more about the differences in cancers between individuals and how to test for these differences to personalize treatment. However, for most cancers, this testing is not part of standard practice.

The side effects of treatment likewise differ depending on the type of chemotherapy and the individual. Two individuals will tolerate the same chemotherapy regimen very differently. Patients may receive the same chemotherapy regimen and one patient will continue working and exercising throughout treatment while the other may experience more fatigue and need quite a bit of rest. The reasons for these different reactions is not clear but is likely related to different genes expressed by the individuals that might play a role in how the body disposes of the particular chemotherapy drugs. Testing for these genes is also in very early stages and is not standard practice for most chemotherapy drugs.

Some side effects are common to all cytotoxic chemotherapy drugs, and some side effects are unique to each individual drug. Most cytotoxic chemotherapy drugs can suppress the bone marrow. As discussed in Chapter 2, the bone marrow is an organ located in every bone in your body. The bone marrow is the factory for making blood cells—the white blood cells, red blood cells, and platelets. After a patient receives chemotherapy, the production of these cells is suppressed and the levels of these cells in the blood decrease. This typically occurs

What is chemotherapy?

10 to 14 days after receiving chemotherapy, and then the bone marrow recovers and the cells return to normal numbers over a period of days. When the white blood cells are low, patients are at risk for infections. When the red blood cells are low, the condition is called anemia, and patients usually feel tired or short of breath. When the platelets are decreased, patients are at increased risk of bleeding. Supportive measures can help offset the lowering of these blood cell levels. Injections can be given to stimulate the bone marrow to produce white blood cells or red blood cells. If the platelets are low enough to significantly increase the risk of bleeding, patients can receive platelet transfusions.

Most cytotoxic chemotherapy drugs can cause some degree of nausea; however, this differs markedly based on the particular drug. With the modern anti-nausea medications, which are given intravenously or in pill form as a preventative measure prior to chemotherapy, nausea and vomiting have become much less common than in the past.

Whether or not a particular chemotherapy drug will cause hair loss or can potentially affect the heart, lungs, kidneys, or liver is dependent on the specific chemotherapy medication. Some chemotherapy medications are associated with diarrhea whereas others are associated with constipation. Supportive medications are available that can improve many of the potential side effects of chemotherapy, and these have made treatment much more tolerable.

See **Table 7-1** for a list of questions to ask your medical oncologist about your chemotherapy treatment.

Table 7-1 Questions to Ask Your Medical Oncologist

What are the names of the chemotherapy drugs I will be receiving?
How often will I receive these medications?
How many treatments equal one "cycle"?
How long will I continue on chemotherapy?
What are the common side effects associated with these medications? Are the side effects temporary or permanent?
How (and when) will I know whether the chemotherapy is working?
What is the goal of the treatment? Is there a possibility that the chemotherapy will cure the cancer, or is the chemotherapy being given to try to keep the cancer under control for as long as possible?

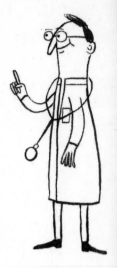

What is chemotherapy?

(Rrest Plate)
Thoracic
(Larynx.
Voice Box,)

Would the CT scan
show Both area's.

CHAPTER 8

What is radiation therapy?

A lot of confusion surrounds peoples' understanding of chemotherapy and radiation therapy. These treatments are quite different from each other. Chemotherapy, as discussed in Chapter 7, is a systemic treatment. Chemotherapy drugs travel in the bloodstream to different parts of the body, the same way that cancer cells can travel in the bloodstream to different parts of the body. That way, chemotherapy can potentially attack cancer cells wherever they might be located in the body. Radiation therapy, on the other hand, is a local treatment. Think about aiming the beam of a flashlight at a part of the body. The light shines only on the particular region of the body where the beam is aimed. Radiation is administered by a machine called a linear accelerator, and the radiation "beam" is aimed at a particular part of the body. Only the tissue in the pathway of this beam is killed. Radiation is one of the two major local treatment options for cancer; the other is surgery. For example, for men with prostate cancer that has not spread beyond the prostate gland, the prostate gland can be surgically removed, or the prostate gland can be irradiated.

Radiation has been used to treat cancer for more than 100 years. Around the time that X-rays were first discovered, they were found to have effects on the body. Many of the early workers with X-rays

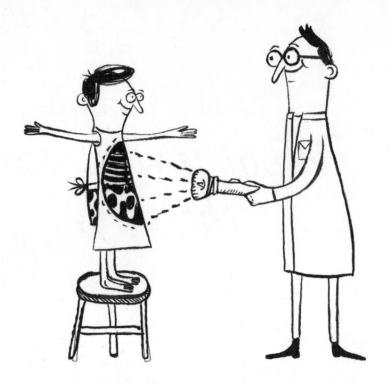

developed redness of their skin in areas exposed to the X-rays. In one of the first experiments attempting to take an X-ray of the skull, the subject's hair fell out. Once it was recognized that X-rays had these effects, Pierre and Marie Curie, the scientists responsible for the major early work with radioactivity, loaned a sample of radium to physicians at a hospital in Paris. The physicians used the radium to try and treat skin cancer and the results were remarkable—the skin cancers in these patients "melted away." Thus, the field of radiation therapy was born. In the early 1900s, Alexander Graham Bell wrote a letter to a physician in New York suggesting that radium could be sealed in a glass tube and inserted directly into a tumor for treatment. This suggestion led to the field of brachytherapy (discussed later).

Radiation therapy actually works in a similar way to chemotherapy by causing damage to DNA, the cells' instruction manual. Although again, unlike chemotherapy in which the medications can travel throughout the body through the blood, the effects of radiation therapy are largely limited to the area at which the beam is aimed. Because the damage sustained from radiation prevents cells from copying their DNA, they cannot grow and divide, and they die. As with chemotherapy, cancer cells are affected to a greater degree than are normal cells because cancer cells are generally growing and dividing more rapidly than normal cells do. In addition, the selectivity of radiation for cancer cells is also based on where the beam is aimed. During the early days of radiation therapy, most of the dose of radiation was administered during one session. Subsequently, it was discovered that giving smaller doses, or *fractions*, over several weeks limits the damage to normal cells and thereby limits the side effects of treatment.

There are two major types of radiation therapy. *External beam* radiation therapy is the most common means of administering radiation. Prior to starting a course of radiation therapy, a radiation oncologist (a physician who specializes in the use of radiation therapy to treat cancer) creates a treatment plan individualized to the specific patient with a procedure called a simulation. In the past, this was done by taking plain X-rays to create a *field* for radiation, or a place to "aim the flashlight," that maximizes the exposure of the cancer to radiation and minimizes the exposure to normal tissue. The reason this is critical is because each normal tissue in the body has a different threshold beyond which radiation will start to cause severe damage to that tissue. In addition, a threshold dose of radiation must be delivered to the cancer tissue to optimize the chances of the radiation

What is radiation therapy?

killing the cancer. It is this balance between maximizing radiation to the cancer and minimizing radiation to the normal tissue that determines the effectiveness and side effects of radiation. With modern-day imaging techniques, this simulation can now be done using a CT scan so that the radiation oncologist can visualize the tumor in three dimensions and use multiple radiation beams that intersect to maximize the radiation to the tumor and minimize the radiation to the normal tissue. Think of placing an orange on a table and having three flashlights shine light on the orange, one from the front and one from each side. The orange will receive much more light than will a plum sitting behind it. Similarly, for example, when irradiating the prostate using multiple beams, the rectum, which sits behind the prostate, can be spared some of the dose of radiation while a sufficient dose to the prostate is still achieved. Newer techniques use a computer to shape the radiation beam and alter the intensity of the beam to further avoid normal tissue. This technique increases the effectiveness of radiation and decreases the potential side effects.

With the simulation, which these days most commonly involves a CT scan, the radiation oncologist maps out the location of the tumor. Then, the doctor works with a physicist and devises a radiation treatment plan that can maximize the dose of radiation to the cancer and minimize the dose to the normal tissue. Sometimes, a body mold or mask is created, which is fitted to the patient. This is done to make sure that when the patient lies on the radiation table each day, there is limited movement so that the same site is irradiated each day. Similarly, a few small permanent tattoo markings, each the size of a mark left by the tip of a pen, are generally placed on the patient's skin to make sure that the patient is in the same position daily. The number of radiation treatments and, therefore, the ultimate dose of radiation depend on the site in the body and the goal of treatment (curative or palliative). However, radiation is most commonly administered once daily, 5 days per week, for 2 to 6 weeks. Each radiation treatment is relatively short, lasting approximately 15 minutes or less. For the treatment, the patient lies down on the treatment table and the radiation therapist makes sure that the patient is in the correct position. Most of the time spent in the treatment room is for positioning. The radiation treatment itself takes only minutes and is painless. However, the machines can be noisy and a bit frightening at first.

Brachytherapy, or internal radiation, involves inserting the radiation source into the body directly near the patient's tumor. By doing this, the tumor receives a large dose of radiation, but the effects on the normal tissue are limited. Generally, a surgeon and radiation oncologist insert the radiation source into the body near the tumor in an operating room. Depending on the type of radiation, the "seeds" or "implants" are removed after a period of time (and a short hospital stay is required), or they are permanent and lose their radioactivity quickly. Internal radiation is commonly used in prostate cancer, cervical cancer, and a variety of other cancers.

Because radiation is a local treatment, the side effects of radiation are generally limited to the site of the body being irradiated. The skin in the field of radiation can be affected, resulting in changes similar to a mild, moderate, or severe sunburn. If the mouth or esophagus is in the field of radiation, temporary damage to the layer of cells that line these organs can result in mouth sores and difficulty swallowing. Radiation to the brain can cause hair loss and nausea. Radiation to the prostate can cause urinary frequency and, sometimes, loose stools. Similar to chemotherapy, the side effects of radiation differ from individual to individual. Side effects from radiation are generally cumulative and may not start until weeks after initiating radiation. Patients who have chemotherapy at the same time as radiation to enhance the effectiveness of the radiation may also experience an increased risk of side effects.

Table 8-1 includes a list of questions to ask your radiation oncologist.

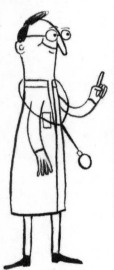

Table 8-1 Questions to Ask Your Radiation Oncologist

How often will I receive radiation treatment?
How many radiation treatments will I receive? How many weeks will my treatment last?
What are the common side effects associated with radiation? Are the side effects temporary or permanent?
How (and when) will I know whether the radiation is working?
What is the goal of the treatment? Is there a possibility that the radiation will cure the cancer?

CHAPTER 9

Why do I have blood drawn at every appointment? What is being tested, and what do the results mean?

Blood tests play a key role in the management of patients with cancer. Through testing of the blood, the treatment team can determine whether the organs are functioning normally and can monitor the effects of chemotherapy on the body. The most common blood test *panels* performed are the CBC, or complete blood count, and the COMP, or comprehensive panel. The results of these tests are generally reported as shown in **Table 9-1**.

Table 9-1 Test Results

Complete Blood Count				
Test	Result	Units	Flag	Reference Range
WBC	9.2	$\times 10^3/\mu L$	Normal	4.8–10.8
RBC	4.43	$\times 10^6/\mu L$	Low	4.5–6.0
HGB	13.7	g/dL	Normal	13.0–18.0
HCT	39.1	%	Normal	39.0–54.0
MCV	88.2	fl	Normal	80.0–100.0
MCH	31.0	pg	Normal	27.0–34.0
MCHC	35.1	g/dL	Normal	32.0–36.0
RDW	14.2	%	Normal	11.0–16.0
PLT	337	$\times 10^3/\mu L$	Normal	150.0–450.0
MPV	7.6	fl	Normal	6.9–10.9
Neu %	93.4	%	High	42.0–71.0
LY %	4.9	%	Low	24.0–44.0
MO %	1.1	%	Low	2.0–12.0
EO %	0.7	%	Normal	0.0–8.0
BA %	0.1	%	Normal	0.0–3.0
Neu # (ANC)	8.6	$\times 10^3/\mu L$	High	2.2–4.8
LY #	0.4	$\times 10^3/\mu L$	Low	1.3–2.9
MO #	0.1	$\times 10^3/\mu L$	Low	0.3–0.8
EO #	0.1	$\times 10^3/\mu L$	Normal	0.0–0.2
BA #	0.0	$\times 10^3/\mu L$	Normal	0.0–0.1

Each blood test is reported with a reference normal range. The normal ranges for blood tests are generally determined by sampling a population of healthy patients to determine the norms. As a result, some patients will have values at the lower end or higher end of normal, but this will be normal for them.

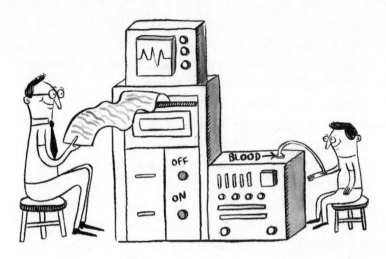

The CBC measures the amounts of blood cells in the bloodstream. Remember from Chapter 2, blood cells are produced by the bone marrow and then are released into the bloodstream. The WBC stands for white blood cell count. The white blood cell count in patients with cancer may be high or low for several reasons. Most commonly, the white blood cell count is low because chemotherapy can temporarily suppress the bone marrow from making new cells. The white blood cell count may be elevated as a result of a medication used to stimulate the bone marrow to make new white blood cells to counteract the effects of chemotherapy; these medications include filgrastim or pegfilgrastim. The white blood cell count may also be elevated as a result of an infection. In patients with cancers of the cells of the bone marrow, leukemia, for instance, the white blood cell count may be elevated as a result of the bone marrow making too many of these abnormal white blood cells.

You will notice that toward the middle of the lab report given in Table 9-1 there is a test result labeled Neu%. All the tests listed from Neu% to the bottom of the report indicate subsets of the white blood cells. The white blood cells come in many different subtypes and each serves slightly different functions in protecting the body from infections and other foreign substances. The Neu% stands for the percentage of the total white blood cell count that are neutrophils. The neutrophils are generally the most important of the infection-fighting cells. Lower down on the report, you will see a test labeled Neu#, also known as the ANC, or absolute neutrophil count. This is a key blood test for patients with cancer who are receiving chemotherapy (and/or radiation). Because the total white blood cell count (WBC) will vary, by knowing the percentage of total white blood cells that are neutrophils, one can calculate the absolute number of neutrophils. For instance, in the lab report, there are 9.2 ($\times$ 10^3/microliter) white blood cells and 93.4% of these are neutrophils. Therefore, the absolute neutrophil count is 8.6 ($\times$ 10^3/microliter). An absolute neutrophil count (ANC) less than 1.0 ($\times$ 10^3/microliter) puts patients at significantly higher risk for developing an infection. Patients who develop fevers when their ANC is less than 1.0 ($\times$ 10^3/microliter) are generally given intravenous antibiotics even if the source of the infection cannot be identified. This is called febrile neutropenia (*febrile* for fever, *neutropenia* for low neutrophil count). The other subsets of white blood cells listed on the lab report include LY (lymphocytes), MO (monocytes), EO (eosinophils), and BA (basophils). There are reasons why any of these subsets can be low or high, but for most patients, the neutrophil count is the most important white blood cell subset to monitor while on chemotherapy.

After WBC on the lab report, you will find a test labeled RBC. All of the tests listed from RBC to RDW are different measurements of the red blood cells. The

RBC test stands for the red blood cell count; however, the HGB (hemoglobin) and HCT (hematocrit) are better tests for monitoring the status of the red blood cells in the body. These tests are generally used interchangeably; some doctors prefer to think in terms of the hemoglobin and others prefer to think in terms of the hematocrit. When the hemoglobin or hematocrit is low, the resulting condition is called anemia. The normal function of the red blood cells is to deliver oxygen to the tissues in the body. So, if the red blood cells are low, there is not enough oxygen being delivered and this manifests in the patient as fatigue, lightheadedness, or shortness of breath. Anemia can result from a multitude of different causes and is very common in patients with cancer. The major causes of anemia include problems with the production of the red blood cells in the bone marrow (for example, when chemotherapy or radiation treatments suppress the bone marrow, or when a patient has a cancer involving the bone marrow such as leukemia), destruction of red blood cells within the bloodstream (for example, as a side effect of certain medications), or loss of blood secondary to bleeding. Anemia can be treated in a variety of ways depending on the cause. Injections called epoetin alfa and darbepoetin alfa can stimulate the bone marrow's production of red blood cells. Generally, when the hemoglobin reaches a level less than 8 g/dL, a blood transfusion is recommended. This cut-off value is somewhat arbitrary and the need for a transfusion will also depend on the symptoms related to anemia and a patient's other medical problems. The MCV (mean cell volume), MCH (mean cell hemoglobin), MCHC (mean cell hemoglobin concentration), and RDW (red blood cell distribution width) are all measurements of different red blood cell parameters that can be useful in determining the cause of anemia.

The PLT blood test is the platelet count. The platelets are the cells in the blood that prevent excessive bleeding. For instance, when you cut yourself, eventually the bleeding stops and a scab forms, which is the work of the platelets. Without platelets, you would continue to bleed and minor cuts and scrapes could be life threatening. The platelet count can be low as a result of several different causes. In patients with cancer, the platelet count is most commonly low as a result of chemotherapy (or radiation) temporarily suppressing the bone marrow from making platelets or from a cancer involving the bone marrow that prevents normal bone marrow function. Platelet transfusions are generally given to patients who are bleeding and have a low platelet count or to patients whose platelet count is lower than 10–20 ($\times$ 10^3/microliter).

A CBC is typically drawn prior to each treatment with chemotherapy. Because chemotherapy can lower the number of blood cells, it is essential to make sure that the blood cells have returned to adequate levels from prior treatment before proceeding with additional chemotherapy. Giving chemotherapy when the blood cell counts are already very low will just cause these cells to drop lower, prolong recovery of the blood cell counts to normal levels, and increase the risk of complications. General guidelines are used to determine whether the blood counts are adequate to proceed with chemotherapy. These guidelines differ somewhat based on the physician, the goal of treatment, and the particular chemotherapy drugs used. Usually, chemotherapy is postponed if the ANC is less than 1.5 ($\times$ 10^3/microliter) or if the platelet count is less than 100 ($\times$ 10^3/microliter). If chemotherapy is repeatedly delayed because the blood counts are low, the dose of the chemotherapy may be adjusted or supportive medications (such as pegfilgrastim) may be added.

The lab report shown in **Table 9-2** is a COMP, or comprehensive panel. This panel of blood tests may go by other names as well, depending on the laboratory.

Glucose is a measure of the level of sugar (glucose) in the blood. The blood glucose may be elevated in patients with diabetes. Alternatively, the value may be elevated in patients receiving steroid medications (such as dexamethasone), which are commonly administered to patients with cancer to prevent nausea and to prevent allergic reactions to chemotherapy, as well as for the treatment of some cancers.

The BUN (blood urea nitrogen) and creatinine values can be used to estimate kidney function. Creatinine is a break-down product of creatine phosphate, which is

Table 9-2 COMP Lab Report

Comprehensive Metabolic Panel				
Test	Result	Units	Flag	Reference Range
Glucose, fasting	225	mg/dL	High	65.0–105.0
BUN	22	mg/dL	Normal	7.0–25.0
Creatinine	1.1	mg/dL	Normal	0.5–1.5
Calcium	9.8	mg/dL	Normal	8.2–10.5
Total protein	6.5	g/dL	Normal	6.0–8.1
Albumin	4.1	g/dL	Normal	3.2–5.0
Globulin	2.4	g/dL	Normal	1.3–3.6
A/G ratio	1.7			
Alkaline phosphatase	91	U/L	Normal	30.0–120.0
SGPT/ALT	19	U/L	Normal	3.0–45.0
SGOT/AST	15	U/L	Normal	3.0–45.0
Total bilirubin	0.4	mg/dL	Normal	0.0–1.4
Sodium	139	mmol/L	Normal	131.0–150.0
Potassium, serum	4.0	mmol/L	Normal	3.5–5.6
Chloride	106	mmol/L	Normal	98.0–114.0
Serum CO_2	24.0	mmol/L	Normal	22.0–31.0

found in the muscles. Creatinine is produced at a fairly constant rate in the body and is filtered through the kidneys. Therefore, rising creatinine levels indicate that kidney function is worsening. The BUN measures the amount of nitrogen in the blood that comes from urea, a waste product made when protein is broken down in the body. A BUN:creatinine ratio greater than 10–20 may indicate that a patient is dehydrated. Kidney function can worsen for several reasons, including dehydration, effects of certain medications (including chemotherapy), contrast dye used for CT scans, and blockage of the kidneys by enlarged lymph nodes, masses, or kidney stones.

The calcium test is a measure of the amount of calcium in the blood. Calcium is essential for the body to function properly. However, too much or too little calcium can be dangerous. A low calcium level in patients with cancer is most often caused by insufficient intake of calcium in the diet. Elevation of the calcium level can occur in patients with cancer that has spread to the bones or as a result of the release of a substance by cancer cells, which causes calcium to be released from the bones into the blood. Manifestations of an elevated calcium level include confusion, nausea, constipation, and a variety of other symptoms. Medications can be given to lower the calcium level in the setting of a dangerously high level.

The total protein, albumin, and globulin are measures of the levels of protein in the blood. The albumin is perhaps the most useful value in the routine monitoring of patients with cancer. A low albumin level generally indicates poor nutrition, which may be the result of a decreased appetite caused by the cancer itself or by cancer treatments.

The alkaline phosphatase, AST (aspartate aminotrans-ferase), ALT (alanine aminotransferase), and total bili-rubin are measures of liver function. An elevation of all of these values generally indicates a problem with the liver or biliary system. However, the AST or ALT may also be elevated transiently as a result of medications that can affect the liver such as certain chemotherapies and Tylenol (acetaminophen), or from other toxins such as alcohol. Alkaline phosphatase can be released from bone, for example, when cancer has spread to the bone. All of these measures can be elevated temporarily from medications; therefore, the trend of the values may be more informative than a single elevated value.

The sodium, potassium, chloride, and serum CO_2 (or bicarbonate) are often referred to as the electrolytes, or "lytes." Electrolytes are generally kept in a normal balance by the kidneys. An elevation or lowering of the electrolytes can be caused by several different processes and results in a variety of symptoms. The electrolytes are routinely monitored in patients undergoing cancer treatment to make sure that these values stay in balance and do not require supplementation.

Some cancers release proteins or other substances into the bloodstream that can be measured with blood tests. These tests are called tumor markers. Unfortunately, most of these blood tests can be elevated by causes oth-er than cancer (with a few exceptions), and therefore, these tests have limited value in diagnosing cancer. Tu-mor markers can be helpful, however, if they are found to be elevated at the time that a cancer is diagnosed. These blood tests can then be measured during treat-ment and used as an indicator of whether the cancer is responding to treatment. Examples of common tumor markers include PSA (for prostate cancer), CA-125 (for ovarian cancer), AFP or alfa-fetoprotein (for liver cancer or testicular cancer), CA 27-29 (for breast cancer), CA 19-9 (for pancreatic cancer), and CEA or carcinoembryonic antigen (for colon cancer, lung cancer, or breast cancer).

CHAPTER 10

Why do I have to undergo all these different types of scans?

Several different types of imaging tests are utilized to generate pictures of the internal organs. Imaging tests are central to the management of patients with cancer. These tests are important in determining whether cancer is localized or whether cancer has spread. In addition, imaging tests allow a determination of whether chemotherapy is effective and a cancer has stabilized or is shrinking, or whether treatment is ineffective and cancer is growing.

Plain films are the general X-rays that you have had in the past and include chest X-rays and X-rays of bones. Although plain films lack the detail of more sophisticated imaging tests, plain films are sometimes the first types of imaging tests that detect an abnormality that leads to the diagnosis of cancer. Furthermore, these films can be obtained and interpreted quickly and are inexpensive compared with newer types of scans.

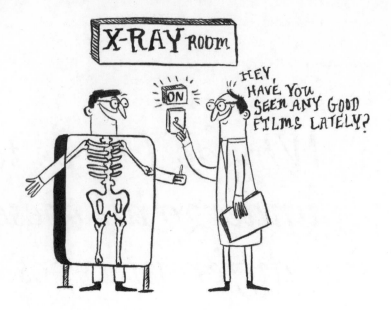

CT scans

Computed tomography (CT) scans used to be called CAT (computed axial tomography) scans. CT scans are generated by a machine that takes a series of X-rays while rotating around your body. The information is then processed (computed) by a computer to produce detailed images of your internal organs.

You can think about the difference between looking at plain X-ray images and CT scan images by imagining a loaf of bread. A plain X-ray image is like looking at the loaf of bread sitting on the table: You can tell it is a loaf of bread, but you can't see a lot of details about the bread. A CT scan image is like inspecting each slice of the loaf separately. Now you can see the full loaf of bread, and also you can see all of the details of the internal aspects of the bread, such as raisins or nuts that it contains. A full CT scan consists of images of the many different slices, just like slices in a loaf of bread, compiled into one scan. For instance, a CT scan of the lungs consists of a series of images taken of the lungs, from the top near the collar bones to the bottom near the abdomen. The following image shows one such slice taken from the series. The black areas are the lungs. The small white lines represent normal markings in the lungs related to blood vessels and airways. However, the larger white mass in the lower right is a lung tumor.

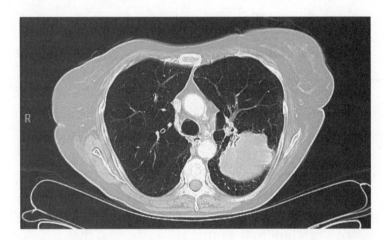

Think about a slice of bread that contains a raisin. When you inspect the individual slice, you can measure the raisin in two dimensions, its height and width. However, to get a real sense of the size of the raisin, you have to look at the adjacent slices of bread to determine whether they also contain pieces of the same raisin so that you can measure its depth. The same is true when looking at CT scan slices. To ultimately determine the size and shape of abnormalities requires looking at slices throughout a region of the body to evaluate the body in three dimensions.

For CT scans, often you will be required to drink oral contrast (a chalky substance) and will be administered intravenous contrast (a substance that is injected into your vein at the time of your scan by a technologist). The purpose of the oral contrast is to opacify (make opaque) your intestinal system so that it can be differentiated from other structures (such as lymph nodes). Similarly, intravenous contrast is administered to differentiate blood vessels from other structures.

When having a CT scan performed, you lie on a table that is then moved through a large round tube called a *gantry*. The length of the exam depends on the parts of the body that are being imaged and typically ranges from about 15 minutes to an hour. During the exam, you may hear the noises of the machine. The exam itself is painless. The technologist sits in the adjacent room and communicates with you via an intercom. The computer generates the images and a radiologist then interprets the exam and generates a report that is sent to your doctor. Risks associated with a CT scan involve exposure to a small amount of radiation and potential allergic reaction to the intravenous contrast dye.

MRI scans

MRI stands for magnetic resonance imaging. MRI scanners produce images that look similar to CT scan images; however, instead of using X-rays to generate the images, the MRI machine uses a magnetic field to create the images. MRI and CT scans can be used to generate images of the same parts of the body; however, MRI scans are preferred in certain locations (such as in the brain) because of the detail they render, and CT scans are preferred in other locations (such as the lungs).

Because MRI scanners use a large magnet to generate their images, patients who have implanted metal objects (such as a pacemaker) should not undergo MRI scans. Similar to CT scans, MRI scans involve lying on a table that is moved slowly into a large hollow tube. With some MRI scans, an intravenous injection of contrast dye is administered. The exam in painless, although some patients feel claustrophobic because of the enclosed space inside the scanner. Newer, more open MRI scanning machines are less confined; however, the quality of the images generated by these machines varies. During the exam, you can hear the machine working, which sounds like loud clunking. The technologist performing the exam stands in another room and communicates with you via an intercom. MRI scans are safe, and as long as you have no implanted metal objects, there are no known harmful effects of exposure to the magnetic field.

Bone scans

A bone scan is in a category of scans called nuclear medicine scans. Nuclear medicine scans involve injection of a small amount of a radioactive material into your body. This material accumulates in different areas of your body and can then be imaged with a special camera called a gamma camera. Depending on the type of radioactive material injected, nuclear medicine scans can be used to detect different types of abnormalities. A bone scan uses a tracer that accumulates in areas in the bone where the cells are very active. Therefore, bone scans can be useful in detecting areas of cancer in the bone but will also detect other causes of abnormal bone cell activity (for example, fractures, infections, arthritis).

Bone scans generate pictures of the skeleton as shown in the following image. The areas that appear dark black are areas where the radioactive tracer has accumulated. This is an example of a normal bone scan. An abnormal bone scan would show dark "dots" in various bones.

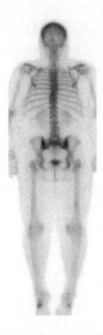

After you are injected with the radioactive material for a bone scan, there is a wait period of a few hours until the material has adequately distributed in your body. During the scan, you lie down on a table and the camera passes over you to take the picture. The images are then interpreted by a radiologist and a report is generated for your physician. Aside from the injection, bone scans are painless. The machine does not involve an enclosed area. The scans take about 30 to 45 minutes. The radiation exposure is negligible.

PET scans

Positron emission tomography (PET) scans are another type of nuclear medicine scan. These scans are used to detect metabolic or chemical activity inside of cells in the body. PET scans require an injection of radioactive material that is similar in structure to chemicals used normally by cells; however, the radioactive material is slightly modified so that it gets trapped inside of the cells. The areas of the body that accumulate the radioactive material can then be imaged with a gamma camera.

The most common PET scans use a radioactive material known as FDG, a sugar-like substance. All cells in your body need sugar to grow, so it makes sense that rapidly dividing cells in your body (such as cancer cells) may use more sugar than normal cells do. PET scans are a relatively new technology, but they have become an integral part of testing for certain types of cancers. PET scans are not used for all types of cancers; for example, cancers that are slowly growing are not well imaged with PET scans. Similar to bone scans, PET scans can also show abnormalities in parts of the body caused by reasons other than cancer. Tissues that are infected or inflamed also use more sugar than normal tissue does and will show up darker on PET scans.

You may be asked to fast or eat a restricted diet prior to your PET scan. After receiving your injection of FDG, you need to wait approximately 1 hour until the tracer adequately distributes throughout your body. The actual scan takes about 30 to 45 minutes. The scan is painless (aside from the injection) and the amount of radiation exposure is negligible.

CHAPTER 11

What are the most important questions I should ask my doctor?

During their training, most oncologists are taught three fundamentals. These principles are simple and might sound a bit obvious. However, doctors constantly reference them to make sure that the treatment of each patient is optimized. These principles also serve as a critical guide for patients who seek to understand their illness and the goals of treatment. You should leave your doctor's office with a clear understanding of the answers to the following questions.

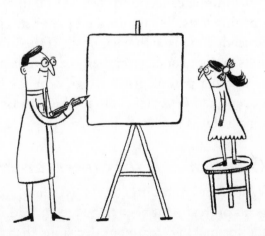

Question 1: Is it cancer?

Not every mass seen on a CT scan or felt on physical examination is cancer. Cancer is a pathologic diagnosis. This means that to make the diagnosis of cancer (with rare exceptions) a sample of tissue must be obtained (a biopsy) and viewed under the microscope. Even biopsies are not 100% accurate. Fine needle biopsies, which remove a very small number of cells from a mass, may be difficult to interpret.

Several years ago, a relative of mine developed an enlarged firm lymph node in his neck. He saw a surgeon, and a needle biopsy was performed. My relative was told that the biopsy results were most likely consistent with head and neck cancer. The pathology slides were reviewed at a major cancer center. The pathologists at that institution thought that the diagnosis was more likely to be lymphoma. A surgical procedure was then performed to remove the entire lymph node. On review of the larger surgical specimen, the pathologist concluded that there was a noncancerous accumulation of white blood cells, but *no* evidence of cancer. This is an unusual situation—most cancers diagnosed as cancer on biopsy are indeed cancer. However, many conditions mimic cancer on physical examination, labs, and imaging tests. Therefore, a biopsy or surgical procedure is needed to make the diagnosis. If the initial biopsy results are not conclusive, then the sample should be sent to another pathologist for review or the biopsy should be repeated. The stakes are too high to assume it is cancer until it is proven to be so.

Question 2: Is the cancer curable?

Whenever cancer treatment is being considered, the goals of treatment need to be recognized. This is essential for making treatment decisions that are acceptable to an individual patient, and it is also important for setting realistic expectations about outcomes. Sometimes the issue of potential curability is not so straightforward. I once saw a patient with a lung mass who on further testing was also found to have a brain mass. Metastatic lung cancer is not considered curable; however, there were some features about the brain mass that were unusual for metastatic cancer. The patient had the brain mass removed surgically, and it turned out to be a benign brain tumor called a meningioma. The lung cancer, therefore, was localized, and the patient was able to have curative surgery. Ask your doctor if your cancer is potentially curable, and if it is not, understand why that is the case.

Question 3: If the cancer is not curable, is it treatable?

There are many reasons to pursue treatment for cancer even if the cancer is not thought to be curable. These include improvement of pain, optimization of quality of life, and prolongation of life. Many diseases in medicine are treated even though the underlying condition is not cured (for example, coronary artery disease or diabetes). With treatment techniques improving, many cancers are being controlled for long periods of time, similar to the model of treatment for these other chronic diseases. If surgery, radiation, or chemotherapy are no longer appropriate, other means of treating symptoms, both the physical and emotional, are available. Even if the cancer is no longer treatable, the patient is always treatable.

CHAPTER 12

My friend says X about cancer. Is it true?

There is a lot of misinformation about cancer. As with many subjects, anecdote sometimes becomes fact and opinion is sometimes favored over scientific data. Most of this misinformation is propagated with the best of intentions. However, the consequences of cancer myths can be quite devastating. Therefore, this chapter dispels some of the more common myths.

Myth 1: Cancer is not curable

Although metastatic cancers, those cancers that have spread to other parts of the body, are not routinely cured, cancers still localized to the organ in which they originated are highly curable with local treatments such as surgery or radiation. Furthermore, progress is being made constantly in an attempt to increase the curability of metastatic cancers. Because progress often moves more slowly than any of us would like, it is easy to lose sight of the major advances that have occurred during our lifetime. For example, in the 1970s a new

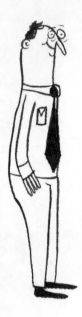

chemotherapy regimen was developed that increased the cure rate of testicular cancers from 25% to more than 80%. Diffuse large B cell lymphoma was once routinely fatal, but with modern treatment approaches, more than 50% of patients are cured of this disease. It is estimated that approximately 80% of childhood cancers are now curable.

Myth 2: Surgery spreads cancer

The myth that surgery results in spread of cancer has been perpetuated for decades. The historical basis for this notion may be the result of poor and unsanitary early surgical techniques. However, just as likely, what was perceived as surgery causing cancer to spread was likely just an observation of the natural history of the cancer. In other words, some cancers behave aggressively. Although scans done prior to surgery may show no evidence that a cancer has spread, cancer cells may have indeed spread long before the surgery but may go undetected on the baseline scans because of their small size. When the patient is "opened up" for surgery, the cancer may be much more extensive than appreciated on the scans performed several weeks earlier. The surgery did not spread the cancer; rather, the lack of resolution on the imaging studies underestimated the extent of the cancer.

Recent laboratory evidence does indicate that surgery may perturb the body and lead to the release of substances that could stimulate cancer growth. However, the significance of these findings in actual patients is unclear. Surgery is the mainstay of curative treatment for patients with localized cancer, and without treatment, these cancers will almost uniformly progress and spread. As a result, the benefits of removing a cancer surgically far outweigh the theoretical risks of surgery promoting its spread.

Myth 3: Chemotherapy causes more harm than good

Chemotherapy is certainly not without a potential down side, and an analysis of the goals of treatment (curative versus palliative) and the possible side effects must be considered for each individual. However, the blanket statement that "chemotherapy causes more harm than good" is often based on anecdotes regarding individual patients who experienced poor outcomes. Often, what is mistaken for side effects of chemotherapy is really a result of the natural history of the cancer in a given patient. For example, patients with advanced cancer who are given chemotherapy may develop progressive fatigue, loss of appetite, and weight loss. However, these symptoms are very commonly associated with progression of the cancer rather than with chemotherapy.

Several clinical trials have shown that in patients with advanced cancer, treatment with chemotherapy can result in an improvement in both quantity and quality of life compared to patients receiving no treatment. In fact, *some* chemotherapy medications were approved by the U.S. Food and Drug Administration specifically because they resulted in an improved quality of life, despite not improving the length of patients' lives. The notion that chemotherapy causes more harm than good is misguided.

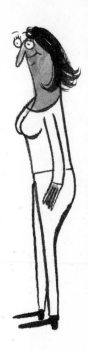

My friend says X about cancer. Is it true?

Myth 4: There is a cure for cancer, but the government, the pharmaceutical industry, and doctors are keeping it a secret

There is no rumor that aggravates cancer doctors more than this one. As previously mentioned, cancers that were not curable 30 years ago are now routinely cured. Advances are made constantly. And, countless friends and relatives of government officials, pharmaceutical industry executives, and physicians have succumbed to cancer. None of these facts is consistent with the hypothesis that the cure for cancer exists, but is being kept secret. In reality, there will likely never be *a* cure for cancer. Cancer is not one disease, but a variety of diseases characterized by different biology. Some cancers have become routinely curable, and with progress, others will become curable as well. The curative treatment regimens, however, will undoubtedly be different for each type of cancer.

Myth 5: Cancer is contagious

You can't catch cancer. You can't pass cancer to your friends and family. Although some cancers are associated with infections (human papillomavirus is associated with cervical cancer), cancer itself is not contagious. You can't pass cancer through sexual intercourse—however, certain infections associated with the development of cancer (again, human papillomavirus is an example) can be passed through intercourse. In addition, barrier protection, such as condoms, are recommended for patients receiving chemotherapy because conceiving a child while undergoing treatment with chemotherapy can be associated with birth defects.

Myth 6: Positive thinking cures cancer

The mind is powerful and can definitely influence physiologic processes in the body. However, there is no evidence that positive thinking can cure cancer. In fact, this issue has been studied in a scientific fashion. In an analysis of more than 1,000 patients with head and neck cancer published in the journal *Cancer* in 2007, the emotional states of patients had no influence on patients' longevity.

I don't bring this up to take away hope. I bring this up because when cancers grow and spread, it is never the fault of the patient for not hoping or wishing hard enough. I have seen blame assigned by friends and family, and blame assigned by patients themselves. Obviously, these feelings are a culmination of guilt and anger and fear, but they are displaced and counterproductive. A positive attitude can help patients comply with treatment and maximize their quality of life.

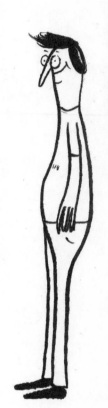

Myth 7: Eating right and taking vitamins can cure cancer

A number of studies have linked certain foods with the development of cancer. However, there is no clear evidence that dietary modifications will cure cancer. Sure, volumes are written on this topic, complete with individual success stories. However, none of these nutritional "cures" have been tested in a scientifically rigorous fashion.

Laboratory evidence shows that high doses of vitamin C may actually promote cancer growth. Remember, cancer cells start as normal cells in the body. They need the same nutrients that normal cells need to grow; however, they typically grow and duplicate much faster than normal cells do. Therefore, they might preferentially absorb the nutrients that they need to grow. A study published in the journal *Cancer Research* in 2008 evaluated cancer cells in the laboratory treated with high doses of vitamin C. The cells were then exposed to a variety of different chemotherapy drugs. The scientists found that the cancer cells that were pretreated with vitamin C grew much faster compared to the cells that had not been pretreated, and all of the chemotherapy drugs were less effective in the vitamin C–treated cells. How these results apply to actual patients is not entirely clear. Nonetheless, given the lack of proven benefit of megadose vitamins, and the potential harmful effects, patients with cancer probably should avoid these supplements, at least while undergoing treatment.

I don't mean to make light of the importance of nutrition. Maintaining a balanced diet and consuming adequate calories are critical while undergoing cancer treatment. Chemotherapy, and cancer itself, can be associated with weight loss, and poor nutrition can be associated with slow recovery and poor wound healing. In addition, certain nutritional exposures (for example, a diet rich in meats high in animal fat or processed meats) likely contribute to the development of certain cancers, and dietary modifications may decrease the risk of developing these cancers. However, for established cancers, eating large quantities of certain foods or supplements is not a secret cure, and maintaining a well-balanced diet is more important.

Myth 8: Eating sugar causes cancer to grow faster

Cancer cells need sugar to grow, just like all cells in the body need sugar to grow. Cancer cells often use more sugar than normal cells do because they are growing faster than normal cells are. In fact, the most common type of PET scan is based on this fact. For an FDG PET scan, a labeled form of sugar is injected into a patient's vein and becomes trapped in cancer cells. A camera can then take a picture of the patient's entire body to pinpoint the sites of highest sugar uptake. This is one test that is used to determine whether a cancer has spread.

The impact of dietary sugar on cancer growth is much more complex than how cancer cells take in injectable sugar. Even if one were to eliminate all sugar from the diet, the body makes sugar from other sources so that it is available to cells. When faced with a diagnosis of cancer, it is still reasonable for patients to limit their intake of concentrated sweets because concentrated sweets raise the level of insulin in the body, which might stimulate cancer growth. A balanced diet consisting of complex carbohydrates, proteins, and unsaturated fats remains the best approach.

CHAPTER 13

I am an individual, not a statistic, so why are clinical trials and their results so important?

Oncology is a data-driven specialty. Because cancer treatments have a narrow therapeutic index (there is a small range between doses that are effective and doses that can cause serious side effects), new cancer treatments must be tested in well-designed clinical trials prior to being accepted as a standard approach.

Phase I, II, and III trials

The development of new drugs for the treatment of cancer generally involves a series of different phases of clinical testing.

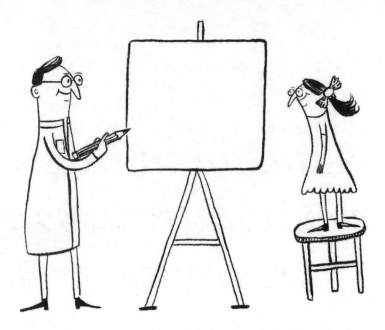

Phase I trials are trials that take a newly developed drug from the laboratory, or a new combination of drugs that have not previously been given together, and test the appropriate dose and schedule of the drug(s) on volunteers. Because these are early trials, generally little is known about the effectiveness of the drugs and the potential side effects. Therefore, only a few patients are treated at a time, and the patients are carefully observed to make sure they experience no severe side effects. If no serious side effects occur, a few more patients are treated using a higher dose, and so on. In this manner, the dose of the drug(s) is increased to a level at which side effects occur that suggest that the drug(s) would not be well tolerated in a large population of patients. The highest dose that does not cause significant side effects is then tested in a phase II trial.

Given that the objective of a phase I trial is to determine the appropriate dose of a new drug or combination, many may wonder why patients would volunteer to participate. Phase I trials do offer several potential advantages. Foremost, these trials are the least restrictive for entry—patients with various types of cancer can enroll, and often there is no restriction on the number of prior chemotherapy treatments. In addition, because these are the newest drugs to be tested, there is always the hope that these novel treatments might be better than the treatments currently available.

In a phase II trial, a group of patients with the same type of cancer are treated with a drug, or combination of drugs, to determine whether the treatment is effective. Phase II trials are usually restricted to patients who have never been treated with chemotherapy, or perhaps those who have received only one prior chemotherapy regimen.

If a drug seems to be effective in a phase II trial, a phase III trial is then performed. Phase III trials involve many patients with the same type of cancer who are randomly selected to join either the group treated with the new treatment or the group treated with the older standard treatment to determine which treatment is better and/ or safer. Phase III trials are generally required for the treatment to gain approval by the Food and Drug Administration (FDA) for standard use in patients.

All of the standard drugs used to treat cancer have undergone a series of clinical trials. New surgical approaches and radiation therapy approaches often proceed through similar phases of testing. Society owes a tremendous debt of gratitude to the patients who volunteered to participate in these trials, without which new treatments for cancer would not exist.

I am an individual, not a statistic

When clinical trials suggest that one treatment is better than another, or that a treatment is better than no treatment at all, statistical testing is involved. Phase III (randomized) trials are required because it is dangerous to rely on anecdotes to treat cancer, such as "My uncle's friend had prostate cancer and went on a grapefruit juice diet for 1 year, and his cancer never spread." Results can happen by chance, and the purpose of a phase III trial is to determine which factor—chance or the treatment under investigation—is responsible for the results. In the example, it is impossible to attribute the fact that the cancer did not spread to the grapefruit juice diet because another factor could have been in effect. For example, *some* prostate cancers do not behave aggressively (in fact, in autopsy studies, about 1 in 10 men has evidence of cancer in their prostate gland although they died of other causes), and this person's case of prostate cancer might have been one such type that would not have spread, grapefruit juice or not. To answer in a scientific fashion whether a grapefruit juice diet can prevent prostate cancer from spreading, a large number of men with prostate cancer would have to be randomized to groups that either follow the grapefruit juice diet or do not. *Randomization* means that a computer decides randomly which patients are assigned to which groups in a controlled experiment—so in this case, which patients would follow the grapefruit juice diet and which patients would not. The reason that randomization is crucial is that without randomization, biases enter the picture that can lead to false conclusions. For instance, if the patients in this trial decided for themselves which treatment they wanted to follow (the grapefruit juice diet or not), one might expect that more health-conscious patients would want to follow the diet. These health-conscious patients may be more likely to follow other healthy practices that might influence the spread of the cancer—for example, they may all take a certain vitamin daily. So, that vitamin supplement may be the real source of the benefit, but the trial would wrongly conclude that the grapefruit juice diet was beneficial. With randomization, *confounding factors* (those factors that are unrelated to the treatment under study but that may influence the results in some way) are usually evenly distributed between the treatment groups. In other words, the number of patients taking the vitamin would be equal in both groups.

Randomized trials must use a large enough sample of patients to make sure that the results of the trials are not from chance and unrelated to the treatment being studied. For example, if you flipped a coin twice and both times that coin landed on heads, you might conclude that the new gloves you were wearing might have caused the coin to land on heads. Of course, this is ridiculous, as the coin landing on heads twice in a row is much more likely the result of chance. On the other hand, if you flipped the coin one hundred times and each time it landed on heads, the probability that this result is related to chance becomes much less likely. Similarly, the larger the number of patients enrolled in a phase III trial, the less likely that the results will be due to chance rather than an actual effect of the treatment under study. Phase III trials typically involve hundreds to thousands of patients.

Statistics in cancer

Interpreting the results of these clinical trials and using these studies to select an appropriate treatment require an understanding of the magnitude of benefit and the potential risks involved with any treatment. As discussed in Chapter 5, some patients with breast cancer (or colon or lung cancer), after surgery, are treated with several months of chemotherapy in an attempt to kill microscopic cancer cells that might have spread even before the surgery. By definition, these micrometastases are microscopic, so there are no tests available to detect them. In an individual patient with no evidence of cancer 10 years after undergoing surgery and chemotherapy, it is impossible to know whether the chemotherapy was necessary to cure that cancer or whether the patient would have been cured with surgery alone. However, multiple phase III clinical trials comparing the treatment of surgery alone to treatment of surgery plus chemotherapy have demonstrated that a higher proportion of women who received both surgery and chemotherapy were alive 10 years later; therefore, *some* of the patients benefited tremendously from the chemotherapy (and would not have been cured with surgery alone).

Some physicians quote these clinical trials, stating that the addition of the chemotherapy decreased the risk of dying from the cancer by 50%. Here is where statistics comes in. This is called *relative risk reduction*, where the percent reduction in events in the treated group is compared to the control group event rate. If the probability of a woman dying from breast cancer after surgery is 2% (in other words, if 100 patients with similar characteristics underwent surgery, approximately 2 would be expected to die from cancer and the other 98 would be cured with surgery), and the addition of chemotherapy decreases the risk of dying by 50%, then instead of 2 out of every 100 women dying of breast cancer, 1 out of every 100 women would be expected to die. This latter number is called the *absolute risk reduction*, which is the difference between the control group's event rate and the experimental group's event rate. This means that 100 women would be exposed to the potential side effects of chemotherapy to benefit 1 of these 100 women. For some patients, this magnitude of potential benefit is not worthwhile enough for them to undergo chemotherapy. If surgery alone was expected to cure only 50 out of 100 patients, and the addition of chemotherapy could decrease the risk of dying by 50%, then an additional 25 patients would be expected to be cured with the addition of chemotherapy. With these odds, most patients would choose to proceed with chemotherapy. From these examples, it becomes clear that using evidence from clinical trials to guide cancer treatments requires an understanding of the magnitude of benefit from treatment and the potential risks of treatment in each individual patient. A one-size-fits-all approach does not work.

One of the most common statistics quoted in the cancer literature is the *survival rate*. This statistic refers to the percentage of patients alive at a given time after the diagnosis of cancer is made. Survival rates have different meanings depending on the population of patients used to generate this statistic and the status of their cancer. For example, for patients with presumed localized cancers who are treated with surgery or radiation with curative intent, the survival rate is generally used to assess the likelihood of curing the cancer. After surgery or radiation for presumed localized cancer, the likelihood that the cancer will recur is generally highest in the first 3 years, and after 5 years the cancer is much less likely to recur. Therefore, *5-year survival rate* is commonly used synonymously with *cure rate*. In reality, late relapses can occur and are more common in some cancers than others. Here is an example to help clarify: Say that the 5-year survival rate for a group of patients with stage II breast cancer is 86%. This means that in a population of 100 women with stage II breast cancer, 5 years from diagnosis 86 patients will be alive and 14 will have died.

Statistics such as these are difficult to apply to individual patients because each individual patient has either a 0% chance of recurrence or a 100% chance. However, considering the probabilities can still be helpful in decision making. Think about those spy movies where the hero is faced with a choice to play Russian roulette for his freedom or be captured. The villain places a loaded gun with six chambers on the table in front of the hero. When the hero is deciding to play the game or not, information about how many of those chambers are filled with live ammunition would be helpful in the decision-making process. Sure, the chance that the gun fires with the first pull of the trigger is an all-or-none phenomenon—it is 0% or 100%. However, the willingness of the hero to play the game could be influenced by the likelihood of the gun firing, which is related to how many chambers contain bullets. The same holds for interpreting risk and probabilities when it comes to deciding about the use of various treatments for cancer. And just as some secret agents would play the Russian roulette game if five out of six chambers had live ammunition, others will only play if only one out of six chambers is filled. As mentioned, these decisions are complex and personal. You and your doctor should have these "choice" discussions.

Survival rates are interpreted somewhat differently in patients with metastatic cancer. These statistics still refer to the percentage of patients alive at a given time after the diagnosis of cancer, though generally, these patients are "alive with disease." For example, a patient with metastatic cancer treated with chemotherapy may experience a shrinkage of her tumor with chemotherapy and a delay in the further growth and spread of the cancer. However, these patients generally require some form of treatment on an ongoing (though sometimes intermittent) basis because the cancer is usually never completely gone. The cancer may be in *remission*, which refers to situations where the cancer has shrunk to the point where it can no longer be seen on conventional scans. The use of survival rates for individual patients with advanced cancer is limited by some of the same difficulties of applying these statistics to patients with presumed localized cancers. The statistics are an average of a large population; plus, they are often based on older data and older treatment methods. Still, probabilities can have some utility in making important decisions regarding treatment and with regard to establishing realistic goals. Knowledge that a clinical trial demonstrated that 30% of patients with metastatic cancer treated with a certain drug were alive 5 years after treatment compared to 15% of patients treated with a different drug can help an individual decide which treatment to pursue, even though these numbers represent averages of outcomes in the patient populations treated with each drug.

I am an individual, not a statistic

CHAPTER 14

What can I do about the side effects of treatment?

Cancer treatment can be associated with unpleasant side effects. Some patients may experience many side effects with a particular drug, or with radiation, and some patients may have minimal side effects. The reasons for these different reactions are not clear and likely have to do with several factors, including differences in the genes involved in metabolizing, or getting rid of, drugs in the body. If side effects develop, patients can take several measures ranging from supportive medications to having the dosage of chemotherapy adjusted to make treatment more tolerable. Optimal symptom management, however, requires regular and honest communication about what you are experiencing with your cancer doctor. If side effects are not being managed effectively, you may have to call your doctor between visits rather than waiting until your next scheduled visit.

The following sections discuss some common side effects of chemotherapy and/or radiation and suggest how to manage them. Obviously, these suggestions are not a substitute for a discussion

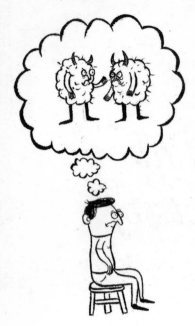

with your doctor but can provide some guidance and support. Your physician and nurse should provide some reinforcement of these chemotherapy teachings. Your likelihood of developing each particular side effect depends in part on the specific drugs you are administered. For example, some chemotherapy medications cause significant nausea whereas others do not. Some medications are more prone to cause constipation whereas others cause diarrhea. Ask your chemotherapy doctor which side effects are most likely to occur from the medications you are receiving. But don't assume you will absolutely experience those side effects.

Nausea and vomiting

Many chemotherapy drugs can cause nausea and vomiting. In doctor-speak, this is referred to as the *emetogenicity* of the drug. The propensity to cause these symptoms differs markedly among drugs. Patients can use different tactics to prevent nausea and vomiting depending on whether the drugs they are receiving are highly, moderately, or only mildly emetogenic. Most nausea associated with chemotherapy occurs in the first 24 hours after treatment. However, some drugs are also associated with delayed emetogenicity, nausea and vomiting that occurs several days after chemotherapy. Specific preventative measures can be used for delayed nausea and vomiting as well.

Prevention of nausea and vomiting has improved markedly since the early days of chemotherapy. Currently, prior to receiving a chemotherapy infusion, patients are given medication to help prevent nausea and vomiting. The medication is usually from a class of medications called 5HT3-antagonists, which block a signal in the brain that causes nausea and vomiting. These medications can be identified because their generic names end in the suffix *–setron*, such as ondansetron, granisetron, and palonosetron. Other medications used to prevent nausea and vomiting are steroid medications (usually dexamethasone) or a combination of steroid and 5HT3-antagonists. Despite these preventative medications, some patients still experience nausea and vomiting. Prior to the start of chemotherapy, patients are usually prescribed medications such as prochlorperazine or metoclopramide to take at home on an as-needed basis if nausea and vomiting should occur. Ask your doctor for a prescription for an anti-nausea medication to have at home, just in case. If nausea and vomiting persist despite these medications, call your doctor. You can try different medications, and you may need an evaluation to rule out other causes of the persistent symptoms.

In addition to preventative medications and as-needed medications for nausea and vomiting, several supportive measures can improve these symptoms such as eating small, frequent meals, avoiding strong odors, drinking lots of water, and avoiding alcohol.

Diarrhea

Chemotherapy or radiation-associated diarrhea can be serious, particularly when it causes the loss of significant fluid and electrolytes and results in dehydration. When untreated, dehydration can lead to a significant lowering of the blood pressure and the need for hospitalization and administration of fluids through an IV. Several supportive measures can control diarrhea and prevent dehydration. These include drinking plenty of fluid (water, juice, or electrolyte-containing sports drinks), avoiding foods and fluids that can contribute to diarrhea (such as milk products), and following a BRAT diet—a diet consisting of *b*ananas, *r*ice, *a*pplesauce, and *t*oast. If your diarrhea is severe or is associated with fevers, cramps, or blood in the stool, you should contact your doctor immediately.

Chemotherapy-associated diarrhea often can be controlled with over-the-counter medications, such as loperamide. However, do not start these medications without first discussing your symptoms with your doctor. When you use these medications, it is critical that you take them correctly; otherwise, they may not be effective. For instance, loperamide is commonly taken as follows: 4 milligrams with the first episode of diarrhea, and then 2 milligrams every 2 hours for the next 12 hours or until the diarrhea is gone (do not exceed 16 mg in a day). Again, prior to starting this medication, discuss it with your doctor and ask for specific dosing instructions. If over-the-counter medications fail to resolve the diarrhea, you can try prescription medications. Regular communication with your medical team is necessary for optimal management of diarrhea, particularly if your symptoms are not improving. At times, the diarrhea is caused by medications other than chemotherapy (for example, antibiotics) and discontinuation of the causative medications is required for improvement.

Constipation

Constipation in patients with cancer may be caused by a variety of factors including chemotherapy medications, narcotic pain medications, and anti-nausea medications. There are several strategies to control constipation, including increasing exercise, drinking plenty of fluids, and increasing dietary fiber (such as eating more fruits, vegetables, and whole grains). When these measures are not effective, over-the-counter medications can help; however, be sure to discuss the symptoms with your doctor before starting these medications. A common "constipation regimen," particularly in patients taking narcotic pain medications, is as follows:

- Docusate—100 milligrams taken three times daily. Docusate helps keep the stools soft so that bowel movements are easier and less painful.
- Senna—2 tabs taken daily. Senna is a mild laxative.

If these medications are ineffective, you can use additional over-the-counter and prescription medications. Call your doctor immediately if you are unable to pass gas, have constipation associated with nausea or vomiting or severe abdominal pain, or have not moved your bowels in 3 days.

Mouth sores

Certain chemotherapy medications and radiation directed at the mouth or throat can cause mouth sores, oral pain, and difficulty eating and swallowing. Measures to improve these symptoms include the following:

- Avoid acidic foods.
- Eat soft foods that are easy to swallow (such as pudding or oatmeal).
- Avoid alcohol-containing mouthwashes.

Frequent mouth rinses with a warm salt water solution can be helpful. When mouth sores are associated with discomfort, you can use a variety of preparations often collectively called "magic mouthwash" or "miracle mouthwash." Some mixtures consist of a numbing medication often combined with bismuth subsalicylate (Kaopectate) or diphenhydramine (Benadryl) solutions. A prescription electrolyte solution mouthwash is also available, which can decrease the risk of developing mouth sores. At times, mouth sores are the result of an infection and can be treated with antibiotics.

Loss of appetite

Loss of appetite may be related to chemotherapy, radiation, other medications, or cancer itself. Loss of appetite may be caused by nausea, a change in taste sensation (a bitter, sour, or metallic taste may occur with chemotherapy; some patients simply notice that everything tastes bland), constipation, or uncontrolled pain. If a single cause for the loss of appetite can be identified, the treatment should be directed at this cause. However, most commonly, there are multiple causes of loss of appetite in a single patient. Some methods of managing loss of appetite include the following:

- Eat small, frequent meals.
- Use calorie supplement "shakes."
- Eat foods with strong flavors (if the problem is that everything tastes bland).
- Use plastic utensils (if the problem is a metallic taste).

In addition to these supportive measures, medications, such as megestrol acetate, can be used to stimulate appetite. If patients are unable to maintain adequate intake of food to reach their caloric requirements, other forms of feeding are sometimes utilized. These include the use of feeding tubes, which allow liquid nutrients to be administered directly into the stomach or intestine, or the use of total parenteral nutrition (TPN), which allows nutrients to be administered intravenously. These alternative forms of feeding are generally used for a short period of time until a patient is able to resume consuming adequate nutrition. For example, a patient who has difficulty swallowing after receiving chemotherapy and radiation for head and neck cancer may receive nutrition through a feeding tube or TPN until his or her swallowing ability returns.

Fatigue

Like many symptoms in patients with cancer, fatigue is often multifactorial. Fatigue may be related to chemotherapy, radiation, pain medications or other supportive medications, infections, dehydration, depression, or other concurrent medical problems. Often, anemia, a lowering of the red blood cells in the body, contributes to feelings of fatigue. Fatigue caused by anemia can be treated with injections to increase the bone marrow production of red blood cells or with blood transfusions.

Some methods of coping with fatigue include the following:

- Take short naps during the day.
- Make sure to drink plenty of fluids.
- Maintain a balanced diet.
- Maintain a light exercise regimen.
- Prioritize activities and ask for assistance with some activities to reserve energy for those that are more important.

Susceptibility to infections

As discussed in Chapter 2, chemotherapy transiently suppresses the bone marrow, the organ located in all of the bones in the body that produces the blood cells. As a result, the number of white blood cells in the blood usually decreases about 10 to 14 days after a patient receives chemotherapy. The degree to which the blood cells decrease depends on the specific chemotherapy drugs and regimen. The bone marrow subsequently can recover and replenish the cells in the blood to normal levels. As mentioned, there are several subtypes of white blood cells. The neutrophils are commonly known as the infection-fighting cells. When the number of neutrophils is low, patients are at increased risk for infections. The infection risk becomes significantly higher when the absolute neutrophil count is less than 1 ($\times$ 10^3/microliter).

When patients develop a fever (generally considered a temperature of equal to or greater than 100.5° Fahrenheit) and the neutrophil count is less than 1 ($\times$ 10^3/microliter), this is called febrile neutropenia. Febrile neutropenia is very serious and requires the urgent administration of intravenous antibiotics (although in some cases antibiotics taken by mouth may be utilized). Patients with febrile neutropenia generally stay on antibiotics until the neutrophil count increases above 1 ($\times$ 10^3/microliter). The neutrophil count also increases as the bone marrow recovers from the effects of chemotherapy; however, sometimes an injection of filgrastim is administered to stimulate the bone marrow in an attempt to speed the recovery. In the majority of cases, the source of the infection is not identified in febrile neutropenia. In fact, most of these infections are probably the result of bacteria that normally live in patients' intestines that transiently gain access to the bloodstream when defenses are down as a result of chemotherapy.

The risk of infections while on chemotherapy may be minimized by following these guidelines:

• Wash your hands frequently.
• Avoid people who are obviously sick.
• Cook food thoroughly.
• Avoid using suppositories when neutrophils are low.

As mentioned, however, the majority of infections in patients on chemotherapy likely come from within the patients' own body, and it is not necessary for patients with solid tumors to quarantine themselves while undergoing chemotherapy. (Patients with liquid tumors, such as leukemia, and patients undergoing bone marrow transplants are different, and these patients often require isolation at times during treatment.) You can minimize the risk of a decrease in your neutrophil count by receiving a shot called pegfilgrastim the day after you receive chemotherapy. The decision to include this shot in a given patient's chemotherapy regimen is based on the likelihood that the neutrophils will drop to dangerously low levels. Your doctor will tell you if you are going to need pegfilgrastim with chemotherapy.

Call your doctor if you experience any of the following while on chemotherapy because these signs and symptoms may suggest an infection:

• Fever of greater than or equal to 100.5° Fahrenheit
• Shaking chills
• Coughing or shortness of breath
• Redness and tenderness at a specific site on the skin

- Redness and discomfort at the site of a port
- Burning with urination

Bruising or bleeding

Another type of blood cell that decreases in the blood after chemotherapy is the platelets. The platelets are responsible for preventing excessive bleeding. The platelet count in the blood will transiently decrease after receiving chemotherapy. The degree to which the platelets decline depends on the specific chemotherapy drugs you are receiving. Most chemotherapy regimens do not lower the platelet count to the range where life threatening bleeding can occur. However, if serious bleeding does occur while patients are on chemotherapy (such as severe blood loss in the stool or coughing up blood), a transfusion of platelets is sometimes required. Platelet transfusions are also commonly given if the platelet count is less than 10–20 ($\times 10^3$/microliter), even in the absence of bleeding, because the risk of major bleeding is significantly increased at these low levels.

Call your doctor if you experience any bleeding while on chemotherapy. Small pinpoint red dots, called *petechiae*, may appear on the skin when the platelets are low; notify your doctor if you develop petechiae.

Hair loss

Hair loss is not universal with cancer treatment and depends on the type of chemotherapy medications being administered or the area of the body being irradiated. Some chemotherapy medications cause hair loss in all patients whereas others are almost never associated with hair loss. Ask your doctor about the likelihood that you will experience hair loss. When hair loss occurs, it typically happens about 3 weeks after the start of treatment. After completing treatment, your hair will start to grow again, although it may take several months before your hair is fully grown.

For some patients, hair loss is one of the more troubling side effects of treatment because it is a constant reminder to patients and others of the presence of the underlying cancer. However, some strategies may make the process of losing hair less devastating. Many patients choose to get a very short hair cut prior to starting treatment to minimize the hair loss that occurs with treatment. Buying a wig prior to starting treatment can be helpful, particularly if you match the wig to your hair color and style. Some patients find wigs uncomfortable and prefer scarves or hats.

Rashes

Several different kinds of rashes can occur in patients receiving cancer treatment. Some rashes are the result of allergic reactions to medications, are side effects of medications, indicate infection, or are reactions to radiation. The treatment of each type of rash is different. You should notify your doctor if you develop a rash.

Numbness or tingling in the fingers and toes

Some chemotherapy medications cause *neuropathy*, damage to the nerves, which results in an abnormal sensation typically in the fingers and toes. The sensation may range from numbness to tingling (like the feeling you get when your foot falls asleep) to a painful sensation. Some patients develop a sensation of walking on sand or with thick socks. Severe neuropathy can cause difficulty walking and difficulty picking up objects or buttoning clothes.

The likelihood of developing neuropathy depends on the specific chemotherapy drugs or regimen in use. When neuropathy initially develops, it may be transient and occur for several days during the chemotherapy cycle and then resolve prior to the next treatment. However, neuropathy can become more constant and even permanent. Notify your doctor if you are experiencing symptoms of neuropathy. To prevent the symptoms from becoming permanent may require a change in the dose of your chemotherapy or even a switch to different medications.

If neuropathy becomes permanent, no medications currently available can cure it. However, some medications available can improve the symptoms of neuropathy, particularly when neuropathy manifests as painful sensations. Medications such as gabapentin and pregabalin, approved by the Food and Drug Administration to treat neuropathic pain, are often used to treat painful neuropathy associated with chemotherapy. Narcotic pain medications are sometimes required if the pain is severe.

CHAPTER 15

I feel like I am going through this alone. Where can I get some help and support?

Cancer can make patients feel isolated. Feeling isolated is a natural reaction to loss of independence and control. No one can truly understand what an individual patient is going through. Despite this, multiple sources of help are available that can help patients cope with the emotional, physical, and financial ramifications of cancer and cancer treatment.

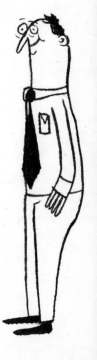

Anxiety and depression are common in patients with cancer, and these symptoms may manifest in several different ways. Feelings of hopelessness and fear may predominate. In some patients, the symptoms may be more physical and include severe fatigue, difficulty sleeping, shortness of breath, and a racing pulse. Tell your doctor if you are experiencing symptoms of anxiety and/or depression. Although these symptoms are a common reaction to cancer

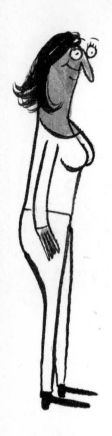

and cancer treatment, the symptoms can also become a problem in and of themselves, interfering with quality of life and compromising treatment. Open communication about these emotions with loved ones and your doctor is essential to coping with these symptoms. Integrative health techniques such as yoga, massage, and other methods of relaxation can be very helpful. At times, anti-anxiety and anti-depressant medications may be needed to manage anxiety and depression optimally.

Many patients take comfort in the fact that multiple other individuals have experienced similar illnesses, treatments, and side effects. Some patients take pleasure in sharing their experiences with patients who are newly diagnosed or who are facing similar treatments in the future. Patients may share means of dealing with certain aspects of cancer treatment that are not always apparent to healthcare professionals. Support groups provide the opportunity for all of these exchanges and can be very helpful in alleviating the fear and anxiety associated with cancer. The different types of support groups range from general support groups open to patients with all different types of cancer, to support groups specific to a particular type of cancer, to virtual support groups on the Internet. Ask your doctor for information about local support groups. Many national cancer advocacy groups have extensive information about particular types of cancer, including information about how to find local support groups. A listing of support and advocacy groups is provided in the appendix.

Some patients experience changes in their functional status as a result of cancer or cancer treatment. These changes may be short term, such as while recovering from surgery or chemotherapy or radiation, or they may be long term. Physical and occupational therapy can be beneficial in terms of speeding recovery, increasing strength, and relearning personal care tasks. Home care with a visiting nurse may be required to more closely monitor ongoing medical problems (for example, wound care) or with a home health aide to help with household tasks. Ask your doctor about setting up these services.

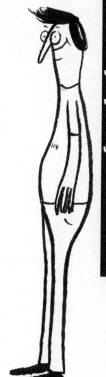

No one wants to think about financial issues when dealing with cancer. However, understanding your insurance plan, including what is and what is not covered, and how much you will need to pay out of pocket can help avoid unpleasant surprises. Prior to undergoing a procedure or initiating treatment, discuss these issues with your insurer. Your doctor's office or hospital may have a financial counselor who can also help you sort through the insurance morass. A social worker can aid in exploring additional means of financial assistance. Many cancer support groups and advocacy groups offer grants to assist with travel, lodging, and coinsurance. Further information about these resources is provided in the appendix.

Appendix

Cancer Advocacy/Resource Organizations

General

American Cancer Society
Telephone: 1-800-227-2345
Web site: http://www.cancer.org

American Psychosocial Oncology Society
Description: Information about local support and counseling services.
Telephone: 1-866-276-7443
Web site: http://www.apos-society.org

Cancer Hope Network
Telephone: 1-877-467-3638
Web site: http://www.cancerhopenetwork.org

Cancer Information and Counseling Line
Telephone: 1-800-525-3777
Web site: http://www.amc.org/counseling/index.html

The Cancer Project
Description: Information on diet/nutrition and cancer.
Telephone: 202-244-5038
Web site: http://www.cancerproject.org

CancerCare
Description: Information and financial assistance for patients
with cancer.
Telephone: 1-800-813-4673
Web site: http://www.cancercare.org

Fertile Hope
Description: Information about treatment-associated infertility
including options for fertility preservation.
Telephone: 1-888-994-4673
Web site: http://www.fertilehope.org

Gilda's Club Worldwide
Telephone: 1-888-445-3248
Web site: http://www.gildasclub.org

Hope Lodge
Description: Assistance with temporary housing for cancer pa-
tients undergoing treatment.
Telephone: 1-800-227-2345 (1-800-ACS-2345)
Web site: http://www.cancer.org/docroot/SHR/content/
SHR_2.1_x_Hope_Lodge.asp

I Can Cope
Description: Education and support for patients with cancer.
Telephone: 1-800-227-2345
Web site: http://www.cancer.org/docroot/ESN/content/
ESN_3_1X_I_Can_Cope.asp

Lance Armstrong Foundation
Description: Information and support for survivors of cancer.
Telephone: 1-866-235-7205
Web site: http://www.livestrong.org

Look Good . . . Feel Better
Description: Program that helps patients with the appearance-
changing side effects of cancer and cancer treatment.
Telephone: 1-800-395-5665
Web site: http://www.lookgoodfeelbetter.org/

National Coalition for Cancer Survivorship
Telephone: 1-888-650-9127
Web site: http://www.canceradvocacy.org

National Lymphedema Network
Telephone: 1-800-541-3259
Web site: http://www.lymphnet.org

National Patient Travel Center
Description: Assistance with medical air travel.
Telephone: 1-800-296-1217
Web site: http://www.patienttravel.org

R. A. Bloch Cancer Foundation, Inc.
Description: Matches newly diagnosed patients with trained
    home-based volunteers treated for same type of cancer.
Telephone: 1-800-433-0464
Web site: http://www.blochcancer.org

Road to Recovery
Description: Assistance with transportation for patients with
    cancer undergoing treatment.
Telephone: 1-800-227-2345
Web site: http://www.cancer.org/docroot/ESN/content/
    ESN_3_1x_Road_to_Recovery.asp

Tender Loving Care
Description: Products for treatments associated with hair loss.
Telephone: 1-800-850-9445
Web site: http://www.tlcdirect.org

The Wellness Community
Telephone: 1-888-793-9355
Web site: http://www.thewellnesscommunity.org/

Bladder Cancer

Bladder Cancer Advocacy Network
Telephone: 1-888-901-2226
Web site: http://www.bcan.org

Brain Tumors

American Brain Tumor Association
Telephone: 1-800-886-2282
Web site: http://www.abta.org

National Brain Tumor Society
Telephone: 1-800-934-2873
Web site: http://www.braintumor.org

Breast Cancer

Breast Cancer Network of Strength
Telephone: 1-800-221-2141
Web site: http://www.networkofstrength.org

Living Beyond Breast Cancer
Telephone: 1-888-753-5222
Web site: http://www.lbbc.org

National Breast Cancer Coalition
Telephone: 1-800-622-2838
Web site: http://www.stopbreastcancer.org

Reach to Recovery
Telephone: 1-800-227-2345
Web site: http://www.cancer.org/docroot/ESN/content/
ESN_3_1x_Reach_to_Recovery_5.asp

Sisters Network, Inc.
Telephone: 1-866-781-1808
Web site: http://www.sistersnetworkinc.org

Susan G. Komen for the Cure
Telephone: 1-877-465-6636
Web site: http://www.komen.org

Childhood Cancer

Candlelighters Childhood Cancer Foundation
Telephone: 1-800-366-2223
Web site: http://www.candlelighters.org

Children's Brain Tumor Foundation
Telephone: 1-866-228-4673
Web site: http://www.cbtf.org

CureSearch
Telephone: 1-800-458-6223
Web site: http://www.curesearch.org

The National Children's Cancer Society
Telephone: 1-800-532-6459
Web site: http://www.nationalchildrenscancersociety.org

Starlight Children's Foundation
Telephone: 1-800-315-2580
Web site: http://www.starlight.org

Colon Cancer

C3: Colorectal Cancer Coalition
Telephone: 1-877-427-2111
Web site: http://www.fightcolorectalcancer.org

Colon Cancer Alliance
Telephone: 1-877-422-2030
Web site: http://www.ccalliance.org

Head and Neck Cancers

The Oral Cancer Foundation
Telephone: 949-646-8000
Web site: http://www.oralcancerfoundation.org

Support for People with Oral and Head and Neck Cancer
Telephone: 1-800-377-0928
Web site: http://www.spohnc.org

Kidney Cancer

Kidney Cancer Association
Telephone: 1-800-516-8051
Web site: http://www.kidneycancer.org

Leukemia and Lymphoma

Leukemia and Lymphoma Society
Telephone: 1-800-955-4572
Web site: http://www.leukemia-lymphoma.org

Lymphoma Foundation of America
Telephone: 1-800-385-1060
Web site: http://www.lymphomahelp.org

Lymphoma Research Foundation
Telephone: 1-800-500-9976
Web site: http://www.lymphoma.org

Lung Cancer

Lung Cancer Alliance
Telephone: 1-800-298-2436
Web site: http://www.lungcanceralliance.org/

Melanoma

Melanoma International Foundation
Telephone: 1-866-463-6663
Web site: http://www.safefromthesun.org

Skin Cancer Foundation
Telephone: 1-800-754-6490
Web site: http://www.skincancer.org/

Multiple Myeloma

International Myeloma Foundation
Telephone: 1-800-452-2873
Web site: http://www.myeloma.org

Multiple Myeloma Research Foundation
Telephone: 203-229-0464
Web site: http://www.multiplemyeloma.org

Ovarian Cancer

National Ovarian Cancer Coalition
Telephone: 1-888-682-7426
Web site: http://www.ovarian.org

Ovarian Cancer National Alliance
Telephone: 1-866-399-6262
Web site: http://www.ovariancancer.org

Pancreatic Cancer

The Lustgarten Foundation for Pancreatic Cancer Research
Telephone: 1-866-789-1000
Web site: http://www.lustgarten.org

Pancreatic Cancer Action Network
Telephone: 1-877-272-6226
Web site: http://www.pancan.org

Prostate Cancer

Man to Man
Telephone: 1-800-227-2345
Web site: http://www.cancer.org/docroot/ESN/content/
ESN_3_1X_Man_to_Man_36.asp

Prostate Cancer Foundation
Telephone: 1-800-757-2873
Web site: http://www.prostatecancerfoundation.org

Us TOO International, Inc.
Telephone: 1-800-808-7866
Web site: http://www.ustoo.org

Thyroid Cancer

Thyroid Cancer Survivors' Association, Inc.
Telephone: 1-877-588-7904
Web site: http://www.thyca.org

I hope this book has addressed your questions—even those you hadn't yet thought of. However, nothing in book form can replace visiting with your doctor, who knows you well.

Index